ETHICAL
DILEMMAS

I dedicate this book to my friend and companion, Linda. Her beauty, patience, and humor enabled me to spend long hours writing, thinking, and musing. Thanks, Love!

GEORGE A. KANOTI

ETHICAL DILEMMAS

A Values Guide for Medical Students

Sage Publications, Inc.
International Educational and Professional Publisher
Thousand Oaks ▪ London ▪ New Delhi

For information:

Sage Publications, Inc.
2455 Teller Road
Thousand Oaks, California 91320
E-mail: order@sagepub.com

Sage Publications Ltd.
6 Bonhill Street
London EC2A 4PU
United Kingdom

Sage Publications India Pvt. Ltd.
M-32 Market
Greater Kailash I
New Delhi 110 048 India

Printed in the United States of America

Library of Congress Cataloging-in-Publication Data

Kanoti, George A.
    Ethical dilemmas: A values guide for medical students / by George A. Kanoti.
        p. cm. — (Surviving medical school; v. 6)
Includes index.
    ISBN 0-7619-1799-3
    1. Medical ethics.   2. Medical ethics—Case studies.   Title.   II. Series.
    R724 .K28 2000
    174'.2—dc21   00-008059

This book is printed on acid-free paper.

00   01   02   03   04   05   06   7   6   5   4   3   2   1

Acquisition Editor:	Rolf Janke
Editorial Assistant:	Heidi Van Middlesworth
Production Editor:	Astrid Virding
Editorial Assistant:	Victoria Cheng
Typesetter:	Tina Hill
Indexer:	Cristina Haley
Cover Designer:	Michelle Lee

Contents

Foreword

During the often hectic and intense years of your clinical training, you will, no doubt, experience ethical dilemmas, complex situations in which responsibility is unclear, emotions are high, stakes are grave, information is inadequate, and moral positions are conflicting. The complexities of such situations, the uncertainty, anxiety, and discomfort they induce, will require your best judgment. How will you prepare?

Ethical Dilemmas, written by one of America's leading medical ethicists, is expressly designed for these difficult choices. First, you will read relevant examples that require you to examine your own beliefs and attitudes, and self-tests will help you address your personal uncertainties and confront moral conflicts. The second section then offers useful guidelines and a procedure for making ethical decisions.

Unique in content and style, this book will appeal to you as a physician-in-training and also to your colleagues who deal with patients in other health care fields.

George A. Kanoti, S.T.D., has more than 20 years of experience as a professor of medical ethics and as a consulting clinical ethicist. After a distinguished university career as professor of theological ethics at the Catholic University of America and Professor of Religious Ethics at John Carroll University in Ohio, in 1980 he established one of the country's first departments of clinical bioethics at the Cleveland Clinic Foundation. Having amassed an impressive wealth of knowledge and experience in teaching clinical ethics to undergraduate, graduate, and health care students as well as to professionals, he has authored articles on clinical and medical ethics in places such as the *Encyclopedia of Bioethics* and the *New England Journal of Medicine.*

His highly interesting book, written in an interactive style, will provide you with invaluable information to enhance your clinical success and personal competence.

—Robert Holman Coombs
Professor of Biobehavioral Sciences,
UCLA School of Medicine
Series Editor

Acknowledgments

The lives, talents, and energies of many persons contributed to this book. Each added color and wisdom to its final form. If there is any value to this work, it is because of them.

I wish to acknowledge a dear friend and mentor, Shattuck Hartwell, Jr., M.D., for his astute and challenging comments on content and form; Claudia Spencer and my son, Byron, for their critical reading and editing; Dorothy Evans who kept me on the right track in the text and disk; and my academic and medical colleagues who stimulated my imagination and extended my knowledge. I give special thanks to the Cleveland Clinic Foundation's bioethicists who shared their rich experiences. Furthermore, I thank the Cleveland Clinic's physicians and surgeons, whose talents and skills gave me health, and the editor of this series, Robert Coombs, Ph.D., who encouraged me to write this volume.

Introduction

"Ed, I am sending you a big problem." Dr. Edward Bronski, the director of the intensive care unit, listens to his ER colleague calmly describe the problem he is passing on. "The patient's name is Wilson Jove, a 32-year-old who crashed his motorcycle early this morning and almost completely severed his left leg at the hip. Before I could stop the bleeding his hematocrit plunged dangerously low. I wanted to give him a blood transfusion. But Jove clearly refused blood because he is a devout Jehovah's Witness. I asked his family for permission, but they also are Jehovah's Witnesses. I gave him some blood expanders, but his condition is very fragile. Good Luck!!"

Dr. Bronski momentarily is angry at the Jehovah's Witnesses because their belief creates a dilemma for him. However, he also knows that making a choice between blood or no blood is filled with agonizing possibilities of physical and psychic injury and guilt to the patient, as well as possible lawsuits and professional scorn for himself. "What are my professional responsibilities?" "What should I do?" "I'm damned if I hang blood; damned if I don't."

Dr. Bronski requests an ethics consultation to help him make a "right" decision. However, the consultation is complicated by confusion over the meaning of words and by strong emotions. *Obligation, duty, law, ethics,* and *morality* are used interchangeably during the discussion of choices. Furthermore, these emotionally charged words evoke contradictory emotions: indignation and resignation ("*I know* what is best for the patient; the law *requires me* to . . ."), guilt and innocence ("*I could not live* with myself if I . . ."; "it is *his* [the patient's] *life* and it is *his choice*"); courage and timidity ("I *willingly* put my reputation on the line by . . ."; "I *fear* the consequences of . . .!"). Conflicting emotions, combined with confusion over the meaning of words, make reasoned thought and discussion very difficult. "What should I do?"

Dr. Bronski's dilemma (which will be discussed in Chapter 3) was my first taste of clinical ethics decision making. This book is the result of years of experience providing clinical ethics advice to physicians, patients, families, and nurses who face "damn situations," in which ethical choices rarely are clear, stress is intense, feelings are conflicted, and professional stakes are high. I have found that clarification of language and concepts is the first step toward good decision making.

Management of feelings is beyond the scope of this book. However, clarification of the words *morality, law, ethics, duty,* and *obligation,* is essential in the study of clinical ethics and clinical ethics decision making. The following definitions will be helpful as you begin this book.

Morality is a collection of cultural imperatives (what you must or must not do). A culture's "morality" is usually found in an oral and/or written collection of moral rules or principles handed down from generation to generation. The Ten Commandments is one example of a collection of moral rules. *Law,* on the other hand, describes the collection of rules and regulations by which a society is governed. Laws can be consistent with morality or go beyond a culture's morality. *Ethics* is the systematic study of morality and the justification for moral rules and regulations. Moral rules may or may not be enforced by society's laws. *Duty* describes a responsibility linked with a specific role. For example, a traffic policeman has a duty to enforce traffic rules. *Obligation* means taking on a responsibility. Signing a loan for an automobile purchase gives you the responsibility (obligation) to pay monthly payments to the lending institution. The above terms are discussed fully in Chapter 4.

This book's intent is to provide both practice guidelines and insight into the methods of resolving medical-ethical questions and dilemmas.

- It is not moralistic because moralizing is often offensive and rarely effective.
- It is not a list of answers to medical ethics dilemmas because even when an ethical dilemma is *definitively* answered, questions persist.
- It does not explore ethical theory because theory rarely is pleasing to the palate.

This book presents practice guidelines and an ethical decision-making model that I developed during my years as a student, teacher, counselor, and clinical ethics consultant. It provides perspective on resolving the complex ethics questions you will encounter in medical training and practice.

1 My Name Is . . .

This book is the product of personal and professional reflection. Because of its personal nature you are entitled to know the intellectual and life journey that undergirds this book. My academic journey crossed lands as diverse and contradictory as the Sahara and the Congo and led to degrees in psychology, philosophy, and Roman Catholic theology. Roman Catholic theology teaches a tight, logical ethics system built on unfailing confidence in the authoritative power of scripture and divinely inspired leaders. Yet, paradoxically, Roman Catholic ethics professors challenge their students to move beyond official norms to probe deeper into the perplexing complexity of behavior and its justification.

My teaching and counseling revealed the practical consequences of following ethical theories and the systems they spawn. Their inadequacies are quickly exposed. Counseling persons who faced ethical choices showed me the harshness of moral systems that impose clear and rigid rules on persons who live in an unclear and contradictory world where moral parameters can shift with the discovery of new knowledge or the impact of social, economic, or political change. While counseling women who had unwanted pregnancies about their moral choices, I saw the chaotic and arbitrary consequences of following rigid philosophical or theological systems that condemned abortions or following moral systems that saw choices as individualized and unique. These women found themselves caught in the middle of a moral and legal debate over the termination of pregnancy that pits "right-to-life" against "freedom-of-choice" proponents. Right-to-life groups regard abortion as morally bankrupt because it takes a human life. Freedom-of-choice proponents stress the uniqueness of each pregnancy and the moral right of a pregnant woman to decide whether to have an abortion. Each claims moral ascendancy, yet neither has dominated the moral terrain. Right-to-life groups see a moral universe in black and white with few shades of gray. Freedom-of-choice proponents have a Technicolor view that allows for individualized expressions of right and wrong. Both views have major limitations. Right-to-life groups are hard-pressed to create a moral solution to reproductive tragedies. Freedom-of-choice proponents turn their heads from the conflict created by individualized moral choices that ignore negative effects on other persons.

Furthermore, years of teaching undergraduate and graduate students have shed light on the importance of ethics in personal and professional life. Students, indeed all persons, need a secure center where their choices and decisions support personal integrity instead of fueling internal conflict and even personal disintegration. The scramble to find direction, security, and certainty is a powerful imperative for action. This inner imperative is perhaps a more powerful motivator for decision and behavior than authoritative pronouncements or legal precedents.

The signature event in my development as an ethicist occurred when I resigned my professorship to undertake the challenges of providing clinical ethics consultation. The move from the quiet reflective university environment to the dynamic clinical world revealed how chaotic and muddled practical ethics decision making can be. Practical ethics decisions are not made in private chambers but rather in open arenas where stresses are great and emotions are high. On my first day in clinic, the following case demonstrated the difference between academic and practical ethics. The case illustrates the problems that physicians face when they must make significant judgments and decisions quickly in unclear or conflicting circumstances.

As I sit at my desk asking myself what, if anything, can I, an academic ethicist, contribute to clinical decision making, my introspection is rudely interrupted by the sharp beep of my newly acquired pager. The summons comes from a pediatric nurse who crisply informs me the chairman of pediatrics requests my attendance at a morbidity and mortality (M&M) conference where a difficult case that "needs ethics input" will be presented. The tone of her voice convinces me that the request is a command. I struggle for questions to identify ethically pertinent information about the death of a three-year-old boy who was being treated on an experimental protocol for a glioblastoma. I mentally identify medical ethics journal references that I want to review to prepare arguments that might make a contribution to the discussion of the case at the M&M conference. When I ask the nurse the date and time of the conference, she says "in 20 minutes."

With clinical ethics decision making, the stakes are high, time is short, and decisions cannot be postponed. As I hurry to the distant room for the M&M conference I collect my thoughts and expect the worst. I learn that the parents' anger at the death of their only son and their implied threat of legal action against the hospital and physician prompted review of the case. When I ask whether the possible lethal side effects of the experimental treatment were discussed with the parents before the therapy was started, the pediatric oncologist responds in an emotionally charged voice, "I was acting in the best interests of my patient!" The physician's evasive answer reveals her deeply held conviction that her duty is to use her knowledge and skills to act for the patient. I see clearly that physicians regard the patient's best interest as a powerful medical ethics norm, a "trump card," that takes precedence over all other considerations, but in this case, the pediatric oncologist's trump card is not balanced by an equally important "wild card," the physician's duty to be honest and thorough when communicating information and options to patients and families. The source of the parents' anger is their perception of a violation of trust. They were not given important information before they consented to the therapy.

Further discussion reveals an important difference between clinical ethics and academic ethics. The physician explains that because the chances of the fatal side effect are statistically so small, she felt she had no duty to reveal the remote possibility of a fatal side effect to already anxious and fearful parents. The physician wanted to avoid alarming the parents, so she merely asked the parents to approve the experimental therapy. The importance of statistical data in medical therapy was not unknown to me, but the power that statistics possesses in clinical ethics judgment and decision making is amazing. This awareness required a 180-degree shift in my own methodology. To communicate effectively with physicians, I needed to provide ethical advice based not solely on abstract ethics principles but also on pertinent statistical evidence and the clinical history of a patient and his or her disease.

This experience taught me important lessons.

- Successful clinical ethics consultation requires a partnership. The ethicist and the clinician must respect each other's knowledge and perspective, and both must focus on the primary goal of clinical practice to discover the option that medically and ethically serves the patient's best interest.

- Physicians can best ascertain what is in their patients' best interest by understanding the patient's personal goals and aspirations.

- Health care professionals carry with them ethical "baggage" that is not exclusively medical in nature. Although each physician is exposed to an ethics "indoctrination" that stresses the physician's duty to use knowledge and power for the good of the patient, each physician carries within himself or herself subtle, yet powerful, moral imperatives and values acquired from ethnic, religious, and political experiences.

- The passage from academia to the world of clinical medicine reveals that although similar interpersonal and intrainstitutional dynamics exist in the medical world as in the academic world, the emphasis is different. In the medical world, power and personality rule rather than suasion and logic.

A Look at the Future

You receive most of your practical clinical ethics training by watching your mentors and teachers handle ethical situations in the examining room, in the office, or during hospital rounds. Fortunately, most of your teachers are responsible practitioners, but you will discover that their ethical advice and skills are limited by their personal moral standards and unique practice. Imitating mentors is effective if you experience similar circumstances when you begin to practice. Unfortunately, you will learn the methods of making ethical choices without formal instruction. You will watch your clinical instructors and mentors make these choices, but rarely will your instructors explain their methods of decision making and the reasons for their ethical choices. This book presents a clinical ethics decision-making model developed through years of observation and practice. Once you have mastered the method, it can assist you as you encounter old and new clinical ethics questions and dilemmas in your practice. You will discover quickly that medical practice in the 21st century exposes you to circumstances that are different from those experienced by your mentors. A subtle change is occurring in the moral ground rules for medical practice that originated in the Western world in the time of Hippocrates. Traditionally, your mentors see their moral duties and responsibilities as rooted in and created by their professional relationship with patients. This one-to-one relationship is the basis for physicians' and patients' moral responsibilities during the relationship. Physicians see their responsibilities and duties to include being loyal to their patients and using their medical knowledge and skills to enhance patients' welfare. In turn, they expect patients to trust them and to "follow the doctor's orders."

Professional and social changes are redefining the physician-patient relationship. The consumer and individual rights movements as well as the introduction of third parties into the patient-physician relationship are changing the moral ground rules. Patients are seeking the best value for their dollar and insisting that physicians respect their right to select or deselect medical therapy. Physicians, in turn, are being pressured to justify both economically and managerially their diagnostic and therapeutic decisions. These and other changes are challenging the traditional moral "certainties" and changing the intellectual and professional preparation for practice in the 21st century.

Furthermore, the introduction of ethicists into the clinical setting has gradually led to the recognition that medical professionals and ethicists can combine intellectual and clinical resources to form a new discipline, "clinical ethics consultation," that brings system and logic to puzzling clinical challenges. This new discipline differs from traditional ethics codes, laws, and judicial precedents.

Clinical ethics consultation addresses perplexing clinical problems by engaging you, hospital administrators, and clinical ethicists in the pursuit of the best solution in contradictory circumstances. Each professional contributes specific carefully honed perceptions, language, and methodologies. The cooperative enterprise demands that you and your colleagues put aside the exclusive language of your tradition and address ethical questions without presumptions built on traditional norms or practice guidelines. Much of this book reflects the cooperative enterprise of clinical ethics consultation in which the exchange of information, theory, and experience contributes to the development of current clinical ethics practice guidelines.

2 To Be or Not to Be a Health Care Professional

Physicians are as different as word processing programs. WordPerfect, WordStar, and the like record ideas and format sentences and paragraphs, but they use different programs to produce the finished document. All physicians diagnose, advise, treat, and follow patients, but each follows a different "program" to fulfill these tasks. These programs (read, styles or methods) in large part reflect their personalities and their values. The following stories describe different styles of communication, making diagnoses, and recommending therapies.

Why Do You Want to Be a Physician?

The Paternalist

> Jamie Price, a coughing and feverish 6-year-old, sits on his family physician's examining table. Angular, gray-haired Dr. Janovich enters the room. Mrs. Price tells Dr. Janovich that the cough and low-grade fever have not improved after 10 days of taking the prescribed cough syrup. He nods his head at Mrs. Price, smiles at Jamie, takes off Jamie's shirt, and places the stethoscope on his chest. Jamie shudders slightly when the cold scope presses against his warm chest. Mrs. Price's terse voice asks, "Could this be something else?" Dr. Janovich, slightly irritated at the interruption, answers in a tone of voice tinged with annoyance. "Mrs. Price, we must let the medicine do its work. Let's give it another week at a higher dosage." His "reas-

suring words" spark a sharp remark from Mrs. Price. "I want another opinion."

Dr. Janovich calls in his new associate, Dr. Rosa, whom Jamie has not met. She is a petite woman with a large smile. She gives Jamie a hug, asks his name, and asks how he feels. "Jamie, please show me where it hurts when you cough." Jamie puts his hand on the right side of his chest. "I am going to listen to your chest now." After warming the stethoscope, she places it on his chest, asks him to cough, and listens intently. Then she turns to Mrs. Price and says she will confer with Dr. Janovich. In a few minutes, Dr. Janovich returns. Dr. Rosa and he do not agree on the cause of the symptoms. Jamie is to be admitted to University Hospital for observation.

Dr. Janovich is an "old school" physician who expects patients to follow his advice. He is kind and considerate but paternalistic in his attitude. He is surprised at Mrs. Price's challenge. Although he is convinced of his judgment, he is willing to consult with a colleague. He honestly admits his disagreement with Dr. Rosa.

He takes charge and begins the process of admission to University Hospital because he believes the admission will assuage Mrs. Price's fears and perhaps prove his own diagnosis is correct. Dr. Rosa, on the other hand, is maternal in her approach. She takes time to introduce herself to Jamie. She hugs him. She asks him questions and warms the stethoscope. However, she does not voice her opinion to Mrs. Price. Dr. Rosa confers in private with Dr. Janovich, gives her opinion, and exits the case.

The Skeptic

Sarah is a doctoral student at a local university. She is unable to concentrate on writing her dissertation because she is experiencing distressing symptoms of low-grade fever and general malaise. She finally makes an appointment with a physician recommended by the nurse in the university's health service office. To her surprise and consternation, the physician, Dr. Van Buren, subtly accuses her of malingering to avoid the onerous task of completing her doctoral dissertation. But despite his veiled accusation, he admits Sarah to the hospital. Dr. Van Buren's attitude toward Sarah changes radically when he enters her hospital room and proudly announces with X ray in hand, "You have an organic disease." Sarah has a blood clot in her lower left lobe.

Dr. Van Buren approaches patients with skepticism. He has treated many university students whose symptoms are due to stress rather than organic disease. Sensitive patients quickly recognize his doubts about an organic cause of their symptoms. He suspects that Sarah is avoiding the task of writing her doctoral dissertation, so his approach to her is tinged with this suspicion. However, when he has scientific "proof" that the symptoms are organic in origin, his attitude changes. He can treat a blood clot! And hopefully, he will find the cause of the clot.

The Scientist

Dr. Sampson enters Mr. Digby's hospital room. Mrs. Digby is seated at the bedside. She has an anxious look on her face. Yesterday, Dr. Sampson told Mrs. Digby that her husband's condition is extremely serious. His liver is failing because of hepatitis B, and his unconscious state is due to hepatic encephalopathy. Dr. Sampson was not encouraging about recovery. Mrs. Digby looks up and begs him to place her husband on the liver transplant list. Sampson gives an ambiguous response. He flips through the patient's chart, examines Mr. Digby, and asks questions of the nurse. As he exits the room he turns to Mrs. Digby and in a tired flat voice says, "Mrs. Digby, my recommendation is your husband should not be treated aggressively. He should be given pain medicine and kept comfortable. Your husband is 70 years old and in the last stages of liver disease. I don't think he is a candidate for a liver transplant."

Mrs. Digby is shocked by his words. Before she can respond, Dr. Sampson leaves the room to see his next patient.

Dr. Sampson presents himself as a "scientific" physician who must make difficult choices based on empirical data. He chooses to ignore the emotional element of Mrs. Digby's plea and addresses her only in scientific and veiled economic terms. He steers clear of conversation with Mrs. Digby and uses the needs of other patients as a justification to shun Mrs. Digby.

Physicians see and interpret clinical ethics questions primarily through the lens of their personal and professional values. Their methods of decision making and conflict resolution reflect their personalities. Unfortunately, few physicians have insight into the role that their values and personality play in their clinical ethics decision making. This lack of self-awareness about the reasons they became health care professionals contributes substantially to the confusion and stress they experience when ethical questions arise in practice.

White coats do not conceal personalities. Physicians' personalities come in all sizes and shapes. There are physicians who are chameleons. They adjust their behavior to reflect each patient's personality whether the patient is a laborer or a corporate executive. Like skilled actors, these physicians interact with their patients to gain their confidence and to discover what each patient wants to hear. Other physicians are as predictable as sunrise. They never vary their approach to a patient. A paternalistic internist remains a paternalistic internist whether he walks into the room of a shy 14-year-old or that of an 85-year-old patrician great-grandmother. Some physicians are direct in their communication of diagnosis and therapy options. Others draw out their patients' feelings and hopes before communicating diagnostic information or therapeutic choices.

The differences in physicians' styles and methods can be traced to a variety of factors, such as philosophic differences in medical school training (e.g., osteopathic vs. traditional medical schools), medical school selection criteria, and so on.

But the most important source of different "bedside manners" is the physician's personality. Despite all the indoctrination and training, physicians rarely alter their personalities during medical school and internship. Just examine your own experience in medical school.

You store and internalize reams of medical information and data. During clinical rotations, you see and practice clinical skills. While you are learning how to practice medicine, you focus primarily on memorizing and regurgitating medical and anatomical information and obtaining approval from your mentors. Internalization and acquisition of skills is influenced deeply by your beliefs, moral values, and goals. Your religious belief or lack of belief, your concepts of right and wrong, and your career goals shape the information and the methods that you learn from your professors and mentors. Your personality and motivation make you a unique person and a unique physician.

The study of clinical ethics is incomplete without discussing personality and motivation. Unfortunately, many medical students are only vaguely aware of what attracts them to a career in health care. The significance of personality and motivation for clinical ethics becomes obvious when questions or dilemmas are faced. Frequently, disagreement or conflict among physicians and between patients (or family members) and physicians occur because their personalities and methods of decision making conflict.

The lack of self-knowledge among candidates for medical careers became evident to me during my tenure as a member of a university undergraduate health care careers committee. Young, eager intelligent students were asked, "Why do you want to become a doctor, nurse, or . . ." Most responses were trite and predictable: "I want to help people"; "I want to find a cure for AIDS." Rarely were the answers personal and reflective. A reflective answer to this question requires that a student move beyond the clichés that readily come to mind. It requires self-awareness and honesty.

Reflective answers reveal a student who brings clarity that will stand him or her well in difficult times. Even the crass and naive response from a brash student, "I want to make money, and medicine seems to be a good way to achieve my goal," gains respect for honesty if not for altruism.

Discussing motivation and personality is a risky business. Personalities and motivations are complicated and complex. It is tempting to repeat offensive stereotypes and create overblown and simplistic caricatures. And yet, examples of motivations provide a chance to see who you are and how others see you.

The Academic Intern

Charlene is an intense young intern who carries in the pockets of her white coat the current issue of the *New England Journal of Medicine* and photocopies of the latest medical news on scientific breakthroughs in medicine. Her quest is to gather as much clinical data as possible so that she can gain insight into the effectiveness of HIV drugs. Most of her time is spent perusing obscure journals and searching the Web for insights and references. She is fascinated by lectures, galvanized by senior physicians' erudite explanations of patients' symptoms, and loves to sit at the feet of the latest medical guru. To Charlene, knowledge is first; patients at best are a means to that knowledge.

The Economic Intern

All of you probably know or will meet Martin. In addition to his stethoscope, Martin carries a palm PC in his lab coat. He is constantly entering data about length of stay, severity of symptoms, number of drugs used per patient, and so on. His fascination is the economics of medicine. Resource allocation, length-of-stay numbers, patient enrollment figures, competition, advertising, and the like capture his attention. To Martin, medicine is a business that requires the skills of an entrepreneur, the focused vision of a CEO, and even, at times, the ruthlessness of a corporate raider. When Martin's senior resident asks him why he would not order a diagnostic test that could reveal the infectious cause of a patient's puzzling symptoms he replies, "The cost of the test is prohibitive and the possibility of meaningful return slight."

His justification for not ordering the diagnostic test reveals how he ranks two very important values: the social value of economy and efficiency over the individual value of patient welfare.

The Star Intern

Almost every medical facility has a Hal. Hal is either a groupie who idolizes the most flamboyant physician or a leader who exhibits narcissistic behavior that attracts those who are inferior in rank. Hal either seeks or fosters "star" qualities: recognition, awe, respect, adulation, and envy. His approach on the wards is signaled by a "buzz," an excitement, among residents, nurses, and students. "The great one is here!"

The Political Intern

The corridors of every hospital have at least one Pauline. Pauline seeks every scrap of gossip about alliances, assignations, ambitions, and so on. Who is sleeping with whom (both metaphorically and physically)? Who are the candidates for head resident? Who is a winner? Who is a loser? Why all this interest in the private and professional lives of colleagues? Because the information may be useful as Pauline maneuvers the maze of the politics of medicine to achieve her goal of position and power.

Self-awareness is the beginning of your training in the art of clinical ethics decision making. A useful way to gain insight into your motivation for pursuing a medical career is to recall the day you realized that medicine is the career you want and to reflect on your feelings about the long and arduous training period. Some persons never doubt that they are destined to be physicians or nurses. No other career attracts them. Others come to medicine along a variety of paths of certainty and uncertainty. They liked their pediatrician; they saw how their parents were deferential to physicians; they may have been born into a family of physicians who assumed that medicine is the only path for their child. Others drift into medicine because of the encouragement and prodding of a teacher or counselor. Self-awareness exposes your moral positions and clarifies your method of arriving at ethical decisions. This clarity illumines the ethical terrain that can contain many pitfalls and booby traps.

Decision-Making Styles

I have witnessed four methods of clinical ethics decision making among health care providers: authoritarian, laissez-faire, scientific, and consensus.

The Authoritarian Approach

This approach relies on the power of the physician's medical knowledge and social role. The physician has all the trappings of authority and power: degree (M.D., Ph.D., MPH, etc.), salutation (this is *Doctor* Jones), dress (lab coat, stethoscope), demeanor (serious, concerned), reputation ("*Doctor* Jones is good. She cured my Johnny's infection"), and so on. All contribute to the perception of power and concern. Usually, patients believe that physicians are acting in their best interest and have more information and experience than they do. Consequently, a firm paternal or maternal direction (aka, prescription) is usually accepted without question.

> "Mrs. Jamison, Billy has an upper respiratory infection. There is an outbreak of these infections in our area. I have treated at least 50 of these infections in the past six weeks. They usually respond to ampicillin. I have written a prescription that should clear up the infection within a week. If there are other problems, or if Billy does not feel better within a week, give me a call."

This physician uses his knowledge and skill to diagnose a problem, prescribe a remedy, and reassure Mrs. Jamison that he will be available if the prescription is not effective or if there is an unexpected negative turn of events. Most clinical education attempts to develop the medical student's confidence in judgment and decision making by challenging a student's intellectual and scientific basis for a clinical decision. As you become more experienced and confident in your diagnosis and therapeutic choices, you will take on the trappings of authority. You become a professional. As one wise physician said, "Doctors may be wrong, but they are never uncertain!"

The Laissez-Faire Approach

The second style, laissez-faire, separates the physician from the duty of making choices. The physician sees his duty to give his patient diagnostic information and therapeutic options. The patient and/or family must make a choice. The physician's duty is to follow the patient's and/or family's choice. In practice, this approach is rarely followed strictly. A laissez-faire physician does not list herbal therapies among the therapeutic options if she does not regard them as scientifically sound, nor does she suggest radical choices like abortion if she is morally opposed to abortion.

> "Mr. and Mrs. Smythe, the tests have returned and show that unfortunately Mr. Smythe's sperm count is very marginal. We have several options that you can choose from. These include adoption, donor insemination, in vitro fertilization, and embryo transfer. Which of these do you wish to pursue?"

This physician gives the Smythes a clear and accurate diagnosis. He also provides them with a menu of the available "therapies"; however, he leaves the choice of therapy entirely up to the Smythes.

The Scientific (Risk/Benefit) Approach

The third style, the scientific or risk/benefit approach, is attractive to physicians who are challenged by the search for answers to incompletely understood disease etiology and the development of more effective therapies. Numbers become normative for their decisions. Human factors, such as patients' preferences, goals, religious beliefs, and so on, do not play a role in decision making. In fact, these factors are seen as distractions and obstacles to be overcome so that patients can agree with the physician's recommendations for the therapy supported by the current scientific and clinical data. The physician's confidence level is usually high. The following conversation between an internist and a patient who has undergone a cardiac angiogram illustrates this style of decision making.

> "Mr. Matthews, I have some good news and some bad news. The good news is we now understand the source of your symptoms. The bad news is that your angiogram shows that your pain very probably is caused by a 50% to 70% blockage in two cardiac arteries. The angiogram also shows that both of these arteries are torturous (twisted) and cannot be opened by balloon angioplasty. I can prescribe medicines to control your chest pain and recommend a rigorous diet, but they probably will not stop the growth of the blockages, nor will these therapies remove the danger of a heart attack. It seems to me that a bypass operation is your best option. Furthermore, in this institution, cardiac bypass surgery is 98% successful in cases like yours. It seems to me that the best choice for you is to undergo surgery. I can schedule your surgery in two weeks."

This style of ethics decision making is powerful and persuasive. The physician presents a diagnosis of the probable cause of the patient's pain and distress based on direct observation through the angiogram. The therapeutic options are clearly presented and are evaluated by using experience and data. Finally, the implicit norm, "this is in your best interest," is used to justify the physician's advice that the patient be scheduled for cardiac surgery.

The Consensus-Building Approach

The fourth style of decision making, the consensus-building method, requires that the physician engage in dialogue with her patient to discover what the patient's expectations are. Then, the physician contributes her judgment about the best therapeutic options. Once this information is on the table, the patient and physician discuss what therapies best "fit" the patient's goals and expectations.

> Dr. Cohen, an oncologist, enters Mrs. Gold's hospital room. She is a 55-year-old woman who is hospitalized for diagnostic testing. "Good morning Mrs. Gold. I hope you had a restful night. I am afraid the re-

sults of your tests are not good. You have an advanced stage of breast cancer. Although it is difficult to predict, this cancer usually moves quickly and is very resistant to conventional therapies. I want to discuss your options with you so you and I can come to an agreement on how to proceed. Among the choices we have are to do nothing except give you pain medication, to give you conventional radiation and drug therapy that has proven about 15% successful in extending life but at great cost of hospitalization and side effects like hair loss and weakness, or to give you an experimental treatment that involves bone marrow transplantation. I am willing to pursue any of these options, but my hope is that you choose the experimental therapy because you are a good candidate. What do you think?"

Mrs. Gold replies, "I have two sons who are engaged to be married in the next three years. One after law school, the other after two years in the Peace Corps. I want to attend their weddings. Let's try the experiment. But Dr. Cohen, if things go bad for me, promise me you will not let me suffer."

The consensus method of decision making is attractive in our culture because Americans value individual choice informed by truthful information. However, the consensus method is rarely practiced in today's hospitals mainly because it is time-consuming and inefficient.

The following questions are designed to structure reflection on your personality, motivation to be a physician, and styles of decision making.

Questions

- When did you become convinced that you wished to become a physician?
- What attracts you to medicine?
- Which stereotype(s) seems to describe your personality?
- What physician(s) do you most admire?
- What characteristic(s) of these physicians attract you?
- Are you more comfortable with the authoritarian, laissez-faire, scientific, or consensus method of decision making?

3 Diagnose Yourself!

Test Your Ethics Decision-Making Skills

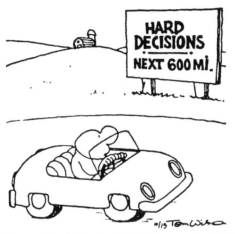

NOTE: *Ziggy* © 1992 Ziggy and Friends, Inc. Reprinted with permission of Universal Press Syndicate. All rights reserved.

What is *responsibility?* The word describes the condition by which you become accountable for your actions or for the welfare of an object, another person, or an organization. For example, in your residency program, you are assigned certain patients for whom you are responsible. You are accountable for these patients. You are required to know your patients' histories, do physical examinations, keep track of all events during their hospital stay, and so on. Failure to meet these requirements brings down the wrath of your immediate superior and the senior physician, especially if your lack of knowledge results in harm to a patient. The ideas of praise and guilt go hand in hand with responsibility. Normally, you receive criticism, or worse, for failure to meet your responsibilities, but rarely are you praised for meeting and exceeding your responsibilities.

Responsibilities arrive wrapped in relationships. All interpersonal and intrainstitutional relationships bring with them expectations, demands, and responsibilities. Your interpersonal relationships begin with total dependence on your mother and others for safety, comfort, and sustenance. These responsibilities are one-way. Your parents and other persons are responsible for you. Over the years, your relationships change from dependent to interdependent relationships and on to an ever-widening web of relationships. Codependent and interdependent relationships bring with them mutual responsibilities.

When you enter medicine, the web of your interdependent and codependent relationships and responsibilities becomes even more complex. In addition to all your other relationships (some active, some inactive, some more active than others), you find yourself making new relationships, encountering new demands, and taking on new responsibilities. The complexity of these relationships and responsibilities frequently creates ethical problems and dilemmas.

The symptom of an ethical problem is well-known. When you ask, "What should I do?" you are facing a choice that involves the question of how to meet a responsibility. The question may be as simple as whether you should do a literature research on the latest AIDS therapy or join your friends at the local pub. Or the question may be as complex as whether you should report a colleague's misbehavior to the authorities. The answer is not always clear.

Problems also arise because either you do not understand or you do not agree with the expectations and assumptions of persons with whom you are in a relationship. Your significant other expects you to spend more time with him or her tonight, but you need to prepare for a comparative anatomy examination. A conflict between choices also may cause problems. You have been advised by your physician to get at least eight hours of sleep each night to reduce stress that is contributing to your persistent upper-respiratory infections. Yet you need an all-night study session to prepare for final exams.

When you walk into an examining room or the hospital room, you carry with you a backpack full of interpersonal and interprofessional responsibilities. Each is clamoring for attention; each claims that you must fulfill it now. What are these responsibilities? You have responsibilities to all of the following: yourself, your significant other(s), your family, your extended family, your colleagues, your patients, their families, nurses and allied health workers, hospital administrators, and finally, the faceless but ever-present law and government.

This chapter presents cases that illustrate problems encountered in clinical practice because of conflicting or uncertain responsibilities. After each case, I offer a brief analysis. This is followed by questions that ask what you think is an ethically acceptable solution to the problem and challenge you to suggest procedures to resolve the case. At the end of the chapter, I present a comprehensive analysis of a case and conclude with recommendations for meeting the responsibilities identified in the case.

Please Help Me!

A low mewing sound seeps out of the half-closed door of a dimly lit hospital room. An intern stands beside the door. Dr. Byrn knows the orders are to give Mrs. Olson pain medicine PRN (as needed) because her metastatic ovarian cancer has moved into her pelvic bones and is causing great pain. She is in end-stage disease. He peers into the room. Mrs. Olson's mouth is a rictus of pain. She looks at him as he prepares to inject morphine into her IV line. "Doctor Byrn, I cannot go on like this. Give me enough to end my misery."

Dr. Byrn shakes his head and says, "Mrs. Olson, I cannot do that. This will make you feel better."

As he turns away, her voice follows him, "Please, please help me." Shaken by his experience and filled with doubts about how he responded to Mrs. Olson's plea for help, Dr. Byrn returns to the on-call lounge. As he enters, he sees a senior physician taking a coffee break.

"Dr. Braun, can I talk to you? Mrs. Olson just asked me to give her an overdose of morphine. I couldn't do it. Should I have given an overdose?"

Dr. Braun stops stirring his coffee, looks up and says, "Welcome to the profession."

Analysis

Dr. Braun's comment exposes the harsh reality of being a physician: Dr. Byrn alone must decide how to use his power and knowledge responsibly. Yet Dr. Byrn feels he is damned if he gives an overdose of morphine to Mrs. Olson because his religious beliefs, as well as current law and professional standards, condemn this action as an act of murder or, at best, assisted suicide. He is damned to doubt and stress if he does not give an overdose because he feels an overdose of morphine would be a medically effective and compassionate way to end Mrs. Olson's pain. Mrs. Olson does not desire to live with the physical pain and the psychic torment of knowing a quick death is possible if only Dr. Byrn would follow her wishes.

Dr. Byrn has an ethical dilemma. Mrs. Olson wants to die. His patient is asking him to help her. His immediate response is to fall back on his professional commitment to "do no harm." His medical training clearly taught him that the ultimate harm to Mrs. Olson is death. And yet, Mrs. Olson is a competent woman who is pleading with him to end her increasing agony. She is in extreme pain. It is her pain. She is in end-stage disease. There is no cure. Pain medications not only dull her pain, they also dull her personality. Is it wrong to end her life mercifully? These doubts lead him to ask an older physician's advice. Unfortunately for him, the older physician only reminds him that the burden of decision is his.

The privileges given to you by society are balanced by the burdens that you assume. Society expects you to use your knowledge and skills to enhance the well-being of your patients. However, exactly what will enhance the well-being of your patient is not always clear. The burden of deciding what is appropriate is yours alone.

Questions

1. What is your personal position on euthanasia and assisted suicide?
2. How did you acquire your position on euthanasia and assisted suicide?
3. How would you respond to Mrs. Olson's request?
4. What reasons support your response to Mrs. Olson's request?
5. Who should make this decision: Dr. Byrn, Mrs. Olson, a judge, Mrs. Olson's family, an ethics committee, other?

To Tell or Not to Tell

3:13 a.m. The ER is quiet. Dr. Andrews stretches and yawns heavily. It is a relatively peaceful Friday night: two heart attacks, a toddler who swallowed a button, one asthma attack, and only one street fight victim. All the patients are successfully stabilized and transferred to other units. His staff is taking an energy break or completing paper work. The peace is broken by an emergency medical service radio transmission announcement that two ambulances are en route to the hospital with three auto accident victims. An elderly couple was returning from their golden wedding anniversary party when a drunk driver ran a red light and crashed into their car. The couple's children came on the scene moments later and called 911 from their car phone. They are accompanying the ambulances to hospital. Their 75-year-old father is in extremely fragile condition; his 70-year-old wife has multiple non-life-threatening injuries. Expected arrival time is 15 minutes. As Dr. Andrews coordinates preparation for their arrival, more details come in. The man's heart is fibrillating. Resuscitation efforts are in progress. The resuscitation is difficult because the patient has extensive chest injuries and loss of blood. His wife has superficial lacerations, a possible concussion, and a broken wrist. She is asking about her husband's condition.

When the ER doors swing open to receive the injured couple, the resuscitation is still in progress. The couple's son-in-law and daughter follow the stretchers into the ER. Dr. Andrews turns to the intern and instructs her to take them to the waiting room until he can report on her parents' condition. After checking the injured wife and directing that she be sent to the trauma center, Dr. Andrews takes command of the resuscitation. He glances at the patient's face and recognizes him. The injured man is Dr. James Wilson. Dr. Wilson is a highly respected physician who served as the county health commissioner until his recent retirement. Minutes later, Dr. Andrews orders a stop to the resuscitation. Dr. Wilson is dead.

As the intern escorts the couples' daughter and son-in-law to the waiting room, Mr. Roberts turns to the intern and tells her, "Doctor, Mrs. Roberts and I agree that you should keep her father's condition from Mrs. Wilson, especially if he dies. She could not handle that information." The intern acknowledges their demand and returns to Dr. Andrews. She conveys the Roberts's demand. Dr. Andrews reports the news of Dr. Wilson's death to the Roberts. They repeat their demand that Mrs. Wilson not be told her husband is dead.

Analysis

Should Dr. Andrews tell Mrs. Wilson the truth or respect her daughter and son-in-law's demand to conceal the truth from her? Three duties are in conflict: respect the wishes of competent patients, tell the truth, and do not harm your patient. Dr. Andrews must decide how to react to the Roberts's demand that the truth be withheld from Mrs. Wilson.

Your relationships with patients carry a responsibility to be truthful to them and to their families. This responsibility is second only to your primary medical duties "do not harm your patients," and "respect the wishes of competent patients." Patients and family members, with rare exception, expect the truth from you. They rely on the truthfulness of your words because your comments structure the confusing reality of illness and injury, and provide light and direction for difficult but necessary decisions. Some of these decisions are literally life and death. Patients and families feel a deep insult if and when they discover that you have not told them the truth.

However, Dr. Andrews is told that telling the truth to Mrs. Wilson will harm her. "She cannot handle" the knowledge that her husband is dead. Dr. Andrews must consider the demands of the children because there may be danger in revealing "bad news" to Mrs. Wilson.

Questions

1. Should Dr. Andrews agree to withhold the truth from Mrs. Wilson?

2. If he agrees to withhold the truth, what should Dr. Andrews say to his staff?

3. If he does not agree with the demand to withhold the truth, how should he convey his disagreement to the Roberts?

4. What should he say to Mrs. Wilson when she asks about her husband's condition?

5. Do you believe that lying to a patient or family member is ever justified? If so, what are your reasons? If not, what are your reasons?

To Treat or Not to Treat?

Dr. Bronski has a splitting headache. Managing the surgical intensive care unit (SICU) is difficult, but cases like this one make him wish he had chosen radiology as his specialty. His staff is divided. The nurses are whispering about what he should or should not do with Mr. Jove's demand. The more callous of the technical support staff are taking bets about whether he will treat. He knows he is damned no matter what he decides to do.

Mr. Jove is a 32-year-old motorcycle enthusiast who suffers a terrible injury. At 2 a.m., his Harley-Davidson skids on wet pavement and crashes into an overpass abutment. His left leg is crushed and almost severed from his torso. He bleeds profusely before help arrives. Incredibly, he is conscious and coherent when the EMS crew arrive. To their astonishment, he tells them that he is a Jehovah's Witness and does not want blood. The crew manages to stabilize him without blood and transport him to the ER. The ER doctors are told the same thing by Mr. Jove, "Do not under any circumstance give me blood! I am a Jehovah's Witness." The ER physicians honor his wishes and use blood expanders to sustain his blood pressure. They treat his most urgent wounds and transfer him to the SICU to prepare for surgery to repair or to amputate his leg.

When Mr. Jove arrives in the SICU, Dr. Bronski speaks with him. Although in pain and groggy from the pain medication, he is coherent and persistent in his demand that he be treated without blood transfusions because he is a Jehovah's Witness. Dr. Bronski reluctantly agrees to respect Mr. Jove's wishes by using more blood expanders and even an experimental blood substitute but with very limited success. Now Mr. Jove's blood pressure is falling slowly, and he is unconscious.

Dr. Bronski wearily moves from his chair into the conference room where Mr. Jove's family is waiting. He meets Mrs. Jove, who is in the seventh month of her third pregnancy. Her two children, ages three and four, Mr. Jove's mother, and several relatives are also in the room. Dr. Bronski soon discovers that all family members are devoted Jehovah's Witnesses. They unanimously support Mr. Jove's rejection of a blood transfusion. Dr. Bronski patiently explains that he has done everything he can to respect their loved one's belief. However, now it is imperative that Mr. Jove be transfused because his blood level is so low that he is unconscious and could easily go into shock and die. A blood transfusion will increase his chances for a good recovery from 5% to 85% or 90%. His arguments and pleas do not alter their position: Do not give him blood. Dr. Bronski's head throbs as he reaches for Tylenol.

Analysis

Dr. Bronski is frustrated and confused. He knows he can prepare Mr. Jove for surgery with a simple standard medical procedure. The blood transfusion would take him to surgery and give him a very good chance to recover even though the recovery would be long and the rehabilitation rigorous. However, competent and seemingly rational persons are thwarting him. They are preventing him from following his medical judgment. Mr. Jove and his family hold a religious belief that in Dr. Bronski's opinion is irrational and potentially lethal. Dr. Bronski has tried all the nonblood products available to him to avoid transfusing Mr. Jove. But Dr. Bronski is losing the battle. The blood expanders and substitutes are not reversing Mr. Jove's downward spiral. What should he do? Continue the present course or give blood?

This case contains a clear conflict between the responsibilities "do no harm" and "respect the wishes of a competent patient" who holds an "unusual belief." If Dr. Bronski respects Mr. Jove's wishes, in all probability he will die. Withholding life-saving therapy from a salvageable patient is an inexcusable breach of his responsibilities. But if he orders a blood transfusion, will his staff obey the orders? What will his colleagues think of his choice? Will the patient and family sue him? Does he have the authority and right to override Mr. Jove's decision? Will the hospital administration support Dr. Bronski no matter what his decision is?

Questions

1. Should Dr. Bronski respect Mr. Jove's wishes and treat him without blood?

2. Does Dr. Bronski have any right to refuse to respect Mr. Jove's wishes?

3. Do you think the duty to respect the freedom of a patient always overrides the duty to save a patient's life?

4. In either case (hang blood or do not hang blood) how should Dr. Bronski address his staff's concerns?

A Family Divided

Mrs. Mancini's condition is worsening. As Dr. Aurelio walks into her room she thinks: "I cannot help liking her." Mrs. Mancini is a tiny but plump 89-year-old widow who is hospitalized for congestive heart failure. Her early Alzheimer's condition makes her warm personality even more attractive. Every day, she greets Dr. Aurelio with a large smile when she enters her hospital room. She makes Dr. Aurelio feel as if she is a new doctor who is going to save her. But her congestive heart failure is worsening. Diuretics and supplemental oxygen are not effective anymore. Her oxygen levels are dropping. She is gasping for breath. Her creatine levels are rising. Placement on a ventilator seems necessary. But Dr. Aurelio is reluctant to order ventilator support because she knows this is the first step in creating Mrs. Mancini's dependency on life support systems that would escalate to placement of a feeding tube and dialysis. All these therapies would delay Mrs. Mancini's death but not prevent it. They would, in fact, prolong her dying.

There is no indication in Mrs. Mancini's medical chart that she prepared any advanced directives. In her present condition, her capability of making rational decisions is out of the question. Dr. Aurelio realizes she must meet with Mrs. Mancini's family to discuss the options. A meeting is arranged with five of her six children. Her sixth child, her youngest, is overseas. The meeting does not proceed well. Her eldest sons, Emilio and Tony, are very emotional. They do not seem to hear Dr. Aurelio's message. They keep saying, "Doctor, you're not giving up on her! You must do everything to make her well." But Gino and Christina tune in to the message and realize that Dr. Aurelio is asking for directions to make decisions about withholding therapy because their mother's condition is irreversible. They try to convey this message to Emilio and Tony, but their conversation turns into a shouting match. Mrs. Mancini's youngest daughter, Gina, seems ambivalent. Dr. Aurelio has to call the meeting to a close.

Analysis

Dr. Aurelio is struggling with the question of whether to begin therapy that will, in all probability, create more harm than good for Mrs. Mancini. Mrs. Mancini has no living will, nor has she appointed anyone as her attorney for health care choices. An informed decision about life support is outside her competence. When Dr. Aurelio turns to the family for guidance, she finds disharmony. She also knows that if this case is scrutinized by the hospital's use-of-resources committee, she would be hard-pressed to justify the use of expensive medical technology in a seemingly futile cause.

Questions

1. Should Dr. Aurelio take on the role of decision maker because there is disunity among the family members?

2. Should Dr. Aurelio start therapy and allow it to run its course?

3. Should Dr. Aurelio make the family vote and follow the majority opinion?

4. What role should economic factors play in Dr. Aurelio's management of this case?

The Whistle-Blower

He did it again. This is the third time Charlie has done it. There it is! Charlie scrawled in Mr. Hughes's chart: "visited patient at 10 p.m. Patient sleeping comfortably. Did visual examination; but did not wake patient." Charlie, Dr. James's fellow, documented that he examined Mr. Hughes at 10:00 p.m. when you know you and he were having a coffee break at 10 p.m. Mr. Hughes is a 40-year-old white male who underwent a successful but difficult cardiac bypass operation five days ago. Because you are a third-year medical student, you diplomatically ask Charlie why he did not check on Mr. Hughes according to the schedule Dr. James ordered. Charlie tells you Dr. James is a new staff physician who is overly cautious. Her orders are unrealistic; besides Mrs. Henry, Mr. Rabinowicz, and Ms. Evans are more in need of our attention. Mr. Hughes is very stable. If anything happens the nurses will page him.

Analysis

The medical student is puzzled and concerned by Charlie's flagrant misdocumentation of activities. Charlie's explanation that other more unstable patients need their attention more than Mr. Hughes seems reasonable. Mr. Hughes is stable, and there seem to be many layers of protection built into the hospital system. Yet Charlie is ignoring Dr. James's order and, more disturbing, he is documenting activities that never happened. The medical student is uncertain about what he should do.

Questions

1. Do you think Charlie made a good clinical decision to devote his time to patients more in need of his attention? Give reasons for your answer.

2. What are the risks of misdocumenting activities in a patient's chart?

3. Does the medical student have a duty to inform Dr. James of Charlie's misdocumentation?

4. Does the role of medical student isolate you from duties and other responsibilities for care of patients?

Walk!! Don't Run!

Your pager buzzes urgently. It signals a cardiac arrest. This is your first code. You look at your resident, Dr. Reston, and ask where the code is located. He glances up from the phone and says, "Oh, it's Mrs. Healy, 300 South." You turn quickly and begin to run toward the stairs. Dr. Reston's sharp voice stops you: "Hey! Walk!! Don't run!" Puzzled, but obedient, you walk quickly down the stairs with Dr. Reston to 300 South. As you descend the stairs, Dr. Reston gives you more detail. "Mrs. Healy is a goner. She is 75 with multiple organ failure. Her family is totally unrealistic about resuscitation and refused to make her DNR (do not resuscitate). We are just pouring money down a black hole by continuing to give her life support. Her physician, Dr. Ramirez, told me to 'slow code her.' So we walk, not run, to this code. If we are lucky she will be gone by the time we get there. Ramirez can honestly tell the family that everything was done." You are startled by this information because only yesterday you were given a briefing by the hospital ethicist on the hospital's DNR policy that explicitly rules out slow codes.

Analysis

This case raises several questions. The "slow code" is a form of deception. The slow code deceives the family into believing that "everything (including resuscitation) has been done" to sustain and to save their loved one's life. Because the physician decides that the family's insistence that "everything be done" is unrealistic and harmful both to the patient and to society, he verbally orders a slow code. In addition, the practice of a slow code creates a dilemma

for the medical student. The medical student sees that he is ordered to participate in a thinly veiled deception that violates hospital policy.

Questions

1. Are you justified in participating in a slow code?
2. Is the deception of slow code justified in this case? Please explain.
3. Do you have any choice but to participate in this slow code?
4. How important are hospital policies concerning resuscitation orders?

Suggestions

Dr. Nevens welcomes you to his seizure service. He mentions that
you have arrived at a very opportune time to witness the use of "suggestions" in making a clinical diagnosis. His announcement intrigues
you because you are interested in the various methods of diagnosing
difficult cases. Furthermore, neurology is the specialty you wish to
pursue. Dr. Nevens explains that one of the most difficult neurological diagnoses is to differentiate the causes of seizures: Are the seizures psychogenic or organic? He describes the patient. Ms. Sally
Lucius is a 33-year-old single woman who has been coming to the
neurology service for two years with complaints of seizures. All attempts to locate the cause of these seizures and to treat them have
proven fruitless. At a recent neurology rounds, his colleagues suggest that perhaps Ms. Lucius is suffering psychogenic seizures or
Munchhausen's syndrome. They recommend using the "suggestion
test." This test involves injecting the patient with a placebo, a saline
solution, and telling the patient that the saline is an active drug that
will produce a seizure. If the patient has a seizure, the cause is very
probably psychogenic. If the patient does not have a seizure, the evidence for an organic cause is strengthened. You accompany Dr.
Nevens into the patient's hospital room and witness the following
dialogue.

Dr. Nevens: "Hello Sally. I have brought a medical student with me
               today. Can I have your permission for her to attend this
               session?"

Ms. Lucius:	"Yes. I want to help students learn. It's the least I can do."
Dr. Nevens:	"Okay. Fine. Sally, I'm going to give you a recently developed diagnostic test to see whether we can find the cause of your seizures and develop a therapy to help you control them. After we connect you to the EEG machine, I will inject you with a drug that will cause you to have a seizure. The EEG will show us where the seizure is located. We will be here to provide help when you have your seizure. Can we proceed?"
Sally:	"Yes."

Analysis

This case raises the question of whether use of deception or lying in clinical practice is justified. The goal of this deception is to arrive at a confident diagnosis that either excludes or includes psychogenic seizure or a possible Munchhausen's syndrome.

Physicians use the patient's description of their symptoms and the history of their illness to start the search for a diagnosis. When patients dissimulate or hide important data, the task of diagnosis becomes very difficult, if not impossible, to complete. These factors, combined with the increasing demand to be efficient and cost-effective, pressure physicians to choose the quickest and most efficient way to make diagnoses. Thus, Dr. Nevens is tempted to use deception.

Questions

1. Is deception justified in this case?

2. What moral and/or legal knowledge is important for making a decision about the ethics of deception in this case?

3. Does the medical student have an obligation to raise questions about the use of the so-called suggestion test?

To Operate or Not to Operate?

Dr. Carter asks you to join him for coffee to discuss a case. His request is unusual because you are an internist and he is a cardiac surgeon. Furthermore, the case does not involve one of your patients. You agree to meet him. He begins the meeting by telling you that he wants your opinion about a patient presented to him for bypass surgery.

Ms. Adams is a 42-year-old woman who has Down syndrome. She has been institutionalized in a state facility since the death of her parents in an automobile crash 30 years ago. She has no living relatives and is a ward of the state. Her parents raised her to be as independent as possible, but she is significantly handicapped. In the state home, she does light chores, such as cleaning and dusting. Staff and patients all like and love her. Recently, she developed symptoms of angina that prompted an exploratory angiogram. The angiogram revealed severe blockages in four cardiac arteries. The cardiologist referred Ms. Adams to Dr. Carter for bypass surgery. Dr. Carter is having doubts about operating on Ms. Adams and wants your opinion.

His doubts are founded on two factors. One is Ms. Adam's reaction to the angiogram procedure, and the other is the justification for performing an expensive operation on a Down syndrome patient. Adam's cardiologist told Carter that Ms. Adams did not comprehend the purpose of the angiogram nor what she was asked to do during the angiogram. Although she was lightly sedated, she became very agitated and combative when the initial "stick" was done. Her agitation was so great that she had to be heavily sedated for the angiogram to proceed. Administrators from the state facility reported to him that Ms. Adams now is very afraid of doctors and very probably would not understand the surgical procedure or the rehabilitation. Carter is also concerned about justifying the expenditure of funds and resources for a person whose life expectancy is limited and for whom the bypass operation would require special nursing and counseling support for an extended period of time. There are many other patients who would profit from a bypass operation and who would live longer and more productive lives.

Analysis

Dr. Carter's doubts about performing a bypass operation on Ms. Adams are grounded in two radically different concerns. He is worried that psychic trauma would be caused by the surgery. He does not wish to cause harm to her. Her previous experience supports this concern. Furthermore, Ms. Adams's reaction to the angiogram suggests that she would not be a cooperative patient and thus would complicate the postsurgery care plan. His second concern is that operating on Ms. Adams may not be justified by an economic and resource allocation analysis. More resources would be used in preparing for the surgery and postsurgery. He wonders whether society would accept the use of this expensive and relatively rare surgery to treat a nonproductive member of society when there are many more potentially productive persons who could profit from the operation and begin to contribute to society once again.

Questions

1. What advice would you give to Dr. Carter?
2. What reasons support your advice?
3. Are there any legal directives for giving therapies to physically and psychically handicapped persons?
4. What would be the proper forum for a discussion of this case? The hospital legal department? A departmental meeting? A special task force? Other?

I Cannot Treat . . .

Mrs. Faith is a wealthy, pugnacious 80-year-old widow who is well-known for her eccentricities. She regards doctors as overpaid, underskilled charlatans. Paradoxically, she seeks doctors' help when she is ill. After visiting a succession of physicians, she is now in your examining room because her stiff knees are causing her so much pain that she has trouble getting in and out of her car. As you approach the examining room, your nurse Jackie emerges with arched eyebrows. "Good luck, Dr. Burt!" she whispers as she passes you.

From the moment you walk into the examining room, the atmosphere is filled with tension and confrontation. "You look pretty young to be a doctor. How long have you been in practice?" "Fix my knees!" "You doctors earn too much money. You should be able to do something for me."

Your explanations about the effects of aging on arthritic knees seem to pass over her head unheard. You ask whether the medicine her previous doctor gave her provided any relief. "Oh, I stopped taking it. I don't want to be drugged."

You tell her bluntly that there are no cures for her condition and no palliation for her symptoms if she does not take her medicine.

Nonetheless she insists that something be done. Just as you are about to offer to transfer her care to another orthopedist, she anticipates your move and says, "Don't you pass me off to someone else. I know you are the best in the city." In desperation, you wonder whether giving her a placebo will have a placebo effect, at least for a short time.

Analysis

Mrs. Faith is a difficult patient. She is skeptical of physicians and yet presents herself when her symptoms prove too much to bear. She is confrontational, acerbic, and noncompliant. Dr. Burt does not want to treat her because she is not cooperative, yet she demands he treat her. He is tempted to try a placebo. If the placebo works, Mrs. Faith will attribute its success to his brilliance as a diagnostician and therapist. She has been known to be very generous to those whom she likes.

Questions

1. Does Dr. Burt have a duty to treat Mrs. Faith?
2. What options does Dr. Burt have?
3. What strategies would you suggest to Dr. Burt?

How to Succeed in Residency

You are lucky! You are the only woman among the four finalists in the race to gain one of the two fellowships in neurology at the prestigious South Hospital where you are completing your residency. The competition is great, and little distinguishes the four finalists. As you assess your chances, anxiety hits you. Although you are in the top 3% of your class, you are an unmarried African American woman in a male-dominated southern hospital. You wonder how the issues of gender and race can help or hurt your chances. You decide to talk about your concerns with Dr. Jobe, the residency director, who makes the final decision about the fellowships. Dr. Jobe is a handsome 42-year-old bachelor. Although there are rumors about his cavalier attitude toward women, he has always treated you with respect.

Dr. Jobe listens intently to your concerns. He assures you that gender and race play no role in the selection process. He compliments you about your work during your recent rotation on his service and smoothly comments on your physical (neat, well groomed), and psychological (compassionate, concerned, a good listener) attractiveness.

Then the conversation segues from your qualifications to questions about your private life. He wonders if you are currently engaged in a serious relationship with anyone. You are not, but you are becoming uncomfortable with the drift of this conversation. Dr. Jobe suddenly tells you, "Dr. Howard, to be frank, Dr. Amah has one of the fellowship positions all but locked up. You and Dr. Owens are neck and neck in the competition for the other position. Is there anything you can do for me that could tip the balance in your favor?" His tone of voice and lascivious smile reveal the meaning of his question.

Analysis

Dr. Howard fears that her gender and race could negatively influence her advancement in medicine. This prompts her request for an interview with the residency director, yet her goals for the interview are not clear. She may want to blunt any subtle negative influence that gender and race could have on the selection process. Also, it is possible that she wants to insinuate a subtle threat of a discrimination charge if she is not selected for the fellowship. To her surprise, Dr. Jobe moves the conversation to an exploration of her personal life. His final question seems to be an invitation to sway his judgment by giving him sexual favors.

Questions

1. Do you think Dr. Howard's request for an interview with Dr. Jobe was wise? If so, why? If not, why?

2. How should Dr. Howard answer Dr. Jobe's last question?

3. Should Dr. Howard report Dr. Jobe's behavior? If so, to whom? If not, why not?

4. Should the hospital have a sexual harassment policy?

The Noble Volunteer

As part of your residency program in neurology, you are required to do research. Fortunately for you, the most prolific clinical researcher in the department has asked you to work on his research team. Its members are studying cellular mechanisms that might contribute to developing a therapy for Parkinson's disease. Part of your research responsibilities includes screening patients for obtaining cellular samples from severely afflicted hands. The research protocol requires that cells be obtained by excising the motor branch of the median nerve in the afflicted hands. Removal of the cells will permanently limit the donor's ability to move the thumb.

You meet with Dr. Alton, a 60-year-old retired biology professor, and his wife. Dr. Alton has been diagnosed with early Parkinson's disease. The protocol is explained with special emphasis on the fact that the donation of his median nerve will permanently limit use of his thumb. Dr. Alton agrees to participate in the research by having the median nerve in his left (nondominant) hand removed. He is aware that his participation in this research will have no benefit to him but may aid future victims of Parkinson's. Mrs. Alton, who is also a university professor, volunteers to serve as an experimental control. She is willing to undergo a biopsy of the motor branch of her normal median nerve in her nondominant hand. Dr. Alton looks at his wife and nods his head as if in approval.

Analysis

Mrs. Alton's volunteering to serve as a control in the experimental protocol is appealing to a researcher because the availability of a normal nerve would make the analysis of the cellular differences in the Parkinson's nerve all the more meaningful. But the biopsy would permanently limit the use of Mrs. Alton's thumb. She seems to understand the implications of the biopsy. The research assistant did not ask if Mrs. Alton wished to volunteer. Her offer is totally unsolicited. Her husband seems to approve of the offer. The researcher is tempted to accept Mrs. Alton's offer to serve as a control in the experiment.

Mrs. Alton's volunteering her healthy thumb for research purposes puts two ethical principles in conflict: the principle of individual freedom (Mrs. Alton's offer is freely made), and do not harm your patient (the biopsy would permanently limit the mobility of Mrs. Alton's thumb). Furthermore, the way the researcher chooses to react to Mrs. Alton's request (rejection, acceptance, ambivalence, etc.) raises serious questions.

Questions

1. Do you believe Mrs. Alton's offer should be accepted or refused?
2. How do you weigh options and values when you make a decision?
3. Is patient freedom more important than patient safety?
4. What other information about Dr. Alton and Mrs. Alton do you think would help you make a decision about accepting or refusing her offer?
5. How would you respond to Mrs. Alton's request?
6. Should Dr. Alton's seeming approval of his wife's offer affect your decision?

God's Miracle?

A family conference is called to discuss discontinuing life support for the Reverend Josiah Reynolds, a 56-year-old fundamentalist minister of a very prominent local African American church. Pastor Reynolds recently had a cardiac transplant followed by infection, severe rejection, several cardiac arrests, periods of anoxia, and multiorgan failure. He is currently receiving dialysis and ventilator support. Neurological assessment concludes that his condition fulfills the clinical definition of brain death. There is no hope for recovery.

At the conference are Pastor Reynolds's wife and several church members. Mrs. Reynolds responds to the diagnosis of brain death by telling a story about Pastor Reynolds's recovery from a coma. Fifteen years ago doctors told Mrs. Reynolds that her husband was "beyond hope" because of pneumonia and kidney failure and requested permission to discontinue life support. Mrs. Reynolds refused because she knew that her husband wanted to live and would not give up. He and she have great belief in the power of divine intervention. Prayers for his recovery were offered at his bedside and in his church. Pastor Reynolds emerged from the coma and was discharged from the hospital. For 15 years, he continued his ministry. Frequently, he used his own experience as an example in his sermons and counseling sessions. No! She will not allow the doctors to discontinue life support. God saved him once; God can do it again. Her comments are enthusiastically endorsed by the church members in attendance.

Analysis

This case presents an example of conflict between religious belief and scientific medicine. Pastor Reynolds's wife and congregation firmly believe that "God will take him when He decides." Mrs. Reynolds will not accept the evidence of brain death. Her belief is strengthened because her husband "was resurrected from the dead by God" 15 years ago. Furthermore, the doctors have been wrong before so why not now! In any event, Mrs. Reynolds believes that her husband's life is in God's hands as long as she can prevent the physicians from removing life support.

Two elements frustrate the physicians. The first is the unusual belief of Pastor Reynolds's wife and parishioners, and the second is the use of scarce resources to sustain the physical life of a clinically dead person. Nurses, technicians, laboratory workers, and respiratory therapists commit their time and energy to what they perceive as a hopeless effort. Intensive care space, high-technology equipment, and other medical supplies are being consumed without apparent justification.

Questions

1. What role, if any, does religious belief play in your career as a physician?
2. Do you believe that sustaining Pastor Reynolds's existence with expensive and scarce resources is justified?
3. How would you react to Mrs. Reynolds's insistence that all life-sustaining technology and nursing support continue at a high level?
4. Is there a compromise you could attempt to work out with Mrs. Reynolds?

The Suspicious Father

Edward's ventilator alarm sounds shrilly. Nurses rush into his room and discover that his ventilator tube is disconnected. Quickly and smoothly Nurse Sadowski reinserts the line into the trachea. Edward does not seem to be in any distress. A quick check of his vital signs indicates that all is well or as well as could be expected. Edward is a 14-year-old cerebral palsy (CP) patient who is severely mentally disadvantaged. In addition to his CP, Edward has chicken pox, adult respiratory distress syndrome (ARDS), pneumonia, and acute renal failure. Edward's long-term prognosis is grim. He may recover from this episode, but Ms. Sadowski knows that he will return to the pediatric intensive care unit (PICU) again and again with recurrences of pneumonia, ARDS, and other problems.

Nurse Sadowski suspects that the ventilator tube was deliberately disconnected. This is the third disconnection in the past two weeks. She knows that Edward's father was visiting his son prior to two of the three events. Soon after he left, the alarm sounded. Ms. Sadowski expresses her suspicion to Dr. Stevens, the director of the PICU. She also tells Dr. Stevens that she and other nurses have witnessed angry conversations between Edward's father and mother. Their tension seems to be centered on the difficulties of day-to-day and long-term care for Edward. The nurses' impression is that Edward's father wants to stop life support measures, but his wife wishes to continue treatment.

Analysis

Dr. Stevens faces several important questions in this case. He is concerned about the cause or causes of the ventilator disconnections. Are they the result of poor nursing care, patient movement, or deliberate act? How can he determine which of the above are true? He knows that Ms. Sadowski's suspicions deserve serious attention, but he does not want to confront Edward's father without hard evidence. Also, he must respond to Ms. Sadowski's concern. To ignore or belittle its importance would be harmful to their working relationship. Yet to take immediate action on this evidence alone would be imprudent.

Questions

1. How would you react to Ms. Sadowski's suspicions?

2. Is the use of life support for Edward justified?

3. How should the PICU staff investigate Edward's father?

Where There Is Smoke Is There Fire?

Dr. Jeris is a primary care physician who has been in private practice for 20 years in a medium-sized manufacturing city in the Northeast. He is a prominent member of the community and has served on the boards of several local businesses. Currently, he is on the board of the In-Line Corporation, an international corporation headquartered in his city. Dr. Jeris has provided medical services to the employees of several large manufacturing companies, including In-Line Corporation, for the past 10 years.

Recently, he joined a university-based network of practitioners that gives him access to the university hospital's resources. This arrangement not only provides backup for his practice but also gives him incentive and opportunity to pursue his interest in the epidemiology and demographics of disease. Taking advantage of the opportunities provided by the university medical network, he has permitted a graduate student, Jane Small, to computerize 20 years of his patient files.

She has created a database that summarizes diagnostic, therapeutic, demographic, and epidemiological factors in each case. Jane will use these data as part of her doctoral dissertation. After six months, Jane has entered approximately 80% of the data. She comes into Dr. Jeris's office with a frown on her face. "Dr. Jeris, I have run some preliminary figures on the data. What I see is a disturbing pattern of leukemia cases occurring in the Arlington section of our county. Actually, the cases seem to be concentrated in a downwind direction from the In-Line Corporation laboratory." She presents the data and outlines the suspect area on the county map. The number and concentration of cases are too striking to ignore. Dr. Jeris quickly sees that the concentration of cases indeed has two common factors: employment at the In-Line laboratory and physical proximity to the laboratory.

Analysis

The research reveals a statistical connection between leukemia and the In-Line laboratory. Although this information is preliminary, it raises serious questions.

Questions

1. Is there a responsibility to disclose this information to health authorities?
2. Does Dr. Jeris have a conflict of interest because of his role as an In-Line Corporation board member and as a provider to the company where the issue of environmental pollution is raised?
3. What would you do if you were Ms. Small?

To Feed or Not to Feed:
That Is the Question

Mrs. Chambers is a 91-year-old woman who has Hodgkin's disease. She is well-known on the ward because of her flinty New England personality and her fierce determinism to be treated as she wants to be treated. During the past week, she has been refusing to eat even though she is capable of swallowing and retaining food. The lack of nutrition is a major concern among the staff physicians, nurses, and residents. She is described by the residents as "MOLT (Mrs. Old and Thin)." Her weight loss is alarming. The prognosis is that she will soon succumb to her Hodgkin's disease unless her nutritional status is bolstered.

You accompany her children, her doctor, Dr. Jones, and his residents as they make a last attempt to encourage Mrs. Chambers to eat. When the group walks into her room, she raises her head and glares. "Oh, I see you are trying to gang up on me. Let me save you the trouble. I don't want to eat. Just give me some water and juices. I know I am going to die. Leave me alone!" She looks each one in the eye and then defiantly turns her head away. She refuses to respond to any further questions or comments.

Dr. Jones shakes his head in frustration. "Mrs. Chambers, we all know how you feel. But we also agree that you have more life ahead of you. We are not sure how much. But it can be quality life with your children and grandchildren. Don't force us to act against your wishes." Mrs. Chambers grunts "Keep away!"

You follow the group as they move to a conference room to discuss the interview. Dr. Jones comes right to the point. "I think we should put in a feeding tube. We may have to restrain her, but she will get the nutrition she needs."

Analysis

Mrs. Chambers's situation represents cases in which the question of nutritional support is the issue. The decision to start, withhold, or discontinue nutritional support creates serious problems in many hospitals. The responsibility to provide food and drink to patients seems to allow for no compromise because food and drink are necessary for living. The responsibility to provide food and drink is perceived as so basic that many physicians, nurses, and family members make no distinction between artificially providing nutrients to patients and hand-feeding them. In fact, the delivery apparatus is called "a feeding tube." Dr. Jones feels Mrs. Chambers's need is so great that it justifies his disregarding her clear refusal.

Questions

1. What is your moral position on providing nutritional support to patients who cannot take nourishment?

2. Does the obligation to provide food and water outweigh the obligation to respect the wishes of a competent patient?

3. Is the description of a nasal/gastric tube or a "PEG" tube as a "feeding tube" an appropriate description?

4. Do you think Mrs. Chambers has any rights?

5. Will Dr. Jones face a lawsuit if he inserts the "feeding tube?"

6. Who should judge Mrs. Chambers's quality of life? Mrs. Chambers? Her children? Dr. Jones? The court?

7. What do you think Dr. Jones should do?

I end this chapter by analyzing a case in detail and making recommendations about fulfilling the responsibilities raised by the case. The case is not very dramatic. In fact, it is as humdrum and banal as the common cold. However, close inspection shows that it raises some delicate questions.

The Smoker?

Dr. White sips steaming coffee to ward off the December chill. As she opens the first patient's file, she is struck by the incongruity of the new patient's name, Colin Sanchez. He is the 7-year-old son of an American Hispanic father and Irish-born mother. Two months ago, he and his recently divorced mother moved from Florida to the upper Midwest. Dr. White wonders how Colin is reacting to this winter's first snow. As an icebreaker, she will ask him whether he has made a snowman. The nurse's interview notes and the patient intake form describe Colin as a quiet, intelligent, and cooperative boy who is experiencing asthmalike symptoms.

Mrs. Sanchez is a naturalized citizen of the United States. She is very cooperative and clear as she answers questions about Colin's medical history and symptoms. Her Irish accent is easy to understand. She made the appointment because his symptoms have flared up and his prescription is almost exhausted. The prescription was written by a Florida pediatrician whom Dr. White met at a medical meeting last fall. "What a small world!" she remarks to herself. The prescription calls for albuterol and cromolyn sodium delivered by inhalers.

Colin's medical history is unremarkable except for his asthmalike symptoms and some early childhood atopic dermatitis that is in complete remission. Colin and Mrs. Sanchez agree that his attacks occur almost exclusively in their apartment and never in school. The nurse notes that Mrs. Sanchez moved to the Midwest to be close to her sisters who live in the suburbs. Mrs. Sanchez also told the nurse that she is dating. One man is a frequent visitor to her apartment, and she sees the relationship as promising. Finally, Colin's health care insurance coverage is through Medicaid.

The odor of stale tobacco smoke twitches Dr. White's nostrils when she enters the examination room. After introductions, she reviews Colin's medical history and symptoms with his mother and him. Their responses are consistent with the intake report and the nurse's notes. Mrs. Sanchez prompts Colin to describe two recent attacks. Both occurred in the evening after he returned to their apartment. His symptoms, satisfactorily relieved by inhalers, include shortness of breath, coughing, audible wheezing, and minor chest tightness. As Dr. White leans forward to listen to Colin's lungs, she notices a pronounced tobacco odor in his hair. Dr. White detects some slight wheezing in Colin's lungs. "Mrs. Sanchez, before I write a prescription, let's talk about what causes Colin's symptoms." Mrs. Sanchez nods approval. Dr. White turns to Colin, "Does cigarette smoke bother you?" Colin is about to answer when his mother gives him a warning look. Dr. White pauses and wonders how to react. Should

she redirect the question to Colin and ask Mrs. Sanchez to allow him
to respond? Or should she drop the question and write a prescription?

Analysis

Dr. White's dilemma is prompted by "ethical moments" in the interview. An
ethical moment is the moment when the question of responsibility occurs.
Usually, an ethical moment is signaled by words such as *should, ought,* and
must that suggest obligation or duty. "Should I do this?" "Must I do that?"
These words create a feeling of urgency and importance that prompts a person
to reflect carefully about his or her obligations or duties before taking action.

Dr. White encounters two ethical moments during this clinical examination.
The first comes when she must decide whether Colin's symptoms warrant a
diagnosis of asthma. Her obligation is to choose a therapy that will treat
Colin's symptoms in a medically effective and fiscally responsible way. The
first step in making this choice is to determine whether Colin's symptoms are
asthmatic symptoms. She decides that the diagnosis of asthma is reasonable
because Colin's history, his symptoms, his physical examination, and his previous prescriptions all fit the diagnosis of asthma. She could prescribe more
effective and expensive asthma drugs. But should she? Colin's symptoms are
relatively minor and effectively controlled by the less expensive drugs. Dr.
White decides Colin is experiencing asthmalike attacks; she responsibly can
write the same prescription for Colin because his present prescription is effective and does not cause side effects.

However, Dr. White also knows she will treat Colin more effectively if she
understands what causes or exacerbates his symptoms. Her decision to ask
a question about exposure to cigarette smoke is based on her conviction that
being a physician means more than dispensing drugs. She believes a physician
must practice preventive medicine because it is more effective and economically responsible to prevent illnesses than to treat them. But the question about
exposure to cigarette smoke that she directed to Colin has created a second
more delicate ethical moment in the nascent relationship. Mrs. Sanchez's signal seems to suggest she that does not want Colin to respond to this question.
Should Dr. White redirect her question to Colin about his exposure to cigarette
smoke, or should she respect Mrs. Sanchez's parental signal and not intervene
with more questions?

On the surface, there seems to be no strong obligation compelling Dr. White
to pursue the question because the prescribed medicine is controlling Colin's

symptoms. On the other hand, if the symptoms are caused by cigarette smoke, control of environmental exposure will be more effective than merely treating his symptoms. Her question to Colin prompted Mrs. Sanchez to give Colin what seemed to be a warning look about answering Dr. White's question. If Mrs. Sanchez or one of her male friends is a smoker, Colin's symptoms could be caused by the cigarette smoke. The possibility that Mrs. Sanchez or one of her male friends is a smoker is strengthened by two pieces of evidence: the reported location of the attacks—in their apartment and never in school—and the stale tobacco odor in Colin's hair. What should Dr. White do? She is dedicated to fostering preventive medicine. How far can she pursue this question without injuring the relationship between Mrs. Sanchez and her? Also, Mrs. Sanchez is not her patient. Does she have an obligation to pursue this question further? She must decide whether to continue her inquiry about the precipitating causes of Colin's asthma or to disregard this line of inquiry and write another prescription for albuterol and cromolyn sodium.

Recommendations

The first step that Dr. White can take to clarify her responsibilities is to acknowledge Mrs. Sanchez's ambiguous signal in words such as, "Mrs. Sanchez, are you comfortable with me asking Colin about exposure to cigarette smoke? I noticed you were surprised by my question." Or Dr. White could be more direct and say, "Mrs. Sanchez, I noticed a cigarette odor when I walked into the room. Has Colin been exposed to tobacco smoke? I ask this because asthma can be caused or made worse by cigarette smoke." Mrs. Sanchez's response to these questions will provide avenues for discussing controlling Colin's symptoms by reducing exposure to cigarette smoke or, if Mrs. Sanchez is a smoker, to discuss whether she wishes to stop smoking. Dr. White will fulfill her responsibility to Colin by prescribing an effective therapy and will also fulfill her responsibility to inform both Colin and Mrs. Sanchez about the role that tobacco smoke plays in Colin's asthma attacks and the means available to help persons "kick the habit" of smoking.

4 How to Resolve Clinical Dilemmas

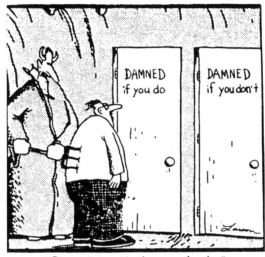

"C'mon, c'mon—it's either one or the other"

Your graduation from medical school will depend in large part on your ability to make responsible choices. Medical education is designed to assist you in perfecting decision-making skills. The medical school faculty members teach you the scientific method of analysis and the results of this analysis. You are expected to understand and retain staggering amounts of scientific information about disease etiology, biology, physiology, and so on. Command of the scientific method and knowledge of scientific findings are important to making diagnostic, prescription, and prognostic choices. However, your decision-making skills are tested in the clinical years through "hands-on" learning. In the clinical years, you are challenged to apply scientific analysis and data to the diagnosis of patients' symptoms and to make decisions about their therapies. Frequently, these decisions have ethical content.

45

Your textbook in the clinical years is the physician-patient encounter. Senior physicians, residents, and fellows are your tutors who show you how they apply scientific inquiry, analysis, and data to the diagnosis of clinical cases. You watch as your tutors take patient histories, perform physical examinations, and communicate their diagnoses to patients and families. You notice that in every clinical workup the moment arrives when therapeutic and/or diagnostic decisions must be made. Frequently, these decisions include ethical questions such as deciding what is best for the patient. For example, should Dr. White (p. 40) renew Colin's prescription or write a prescription for a more expensive medicine? Or what is your obligation to pursue one course of inquiry or another. Should Dr. White raise the question about Colin's exposure to cigarette smoke or merely rewrite the prescription? The clinical years are designed to prepare you to make such decisions.

Unfortunately, the methods of making clinical ethics decisions are rarely taught during the clinical years. In fact, most of your tutors merely draw on their own experiences as medical students, residents, and practitioners, as well as their moral convictions, to develop the personalized style of ethics decision making that you witness during clinical encounters. They rely on these decision-making styles to make decisions in specific clinical circumstances, such as whether to tell the wife of a recently diagnosed HIV patient that her husband has AIDS, how to respond to an angry patient's demands for nonconventional therapy, whether to disclose the diagnosis of severe cardiac arrhythmia to the employer of a 60-year-old school bus driver, whether to continue or discontinue ventilation therapy for an end-stage cancer patient. You watch senior physicians, fellows, and residents making clinical ethical decisions. They, in turn, challenge you to make and defend clinical judgments and propose ethical solutions, and eventually, they expect you to teach others how to make clinical ethical choices.

A Clinical Ethics Decision Model

The clinical ethics decision-making model presented in this book does not require knowledge of ethical theory. However, it does require awareness of your moral convictions (aka, moral knowledge). Chapter 3 is designed to help you uncover your moral knowledge and your personal convictions about right and wrong medical decisions. This chapter presents a decision-making model. A glossary of terms is included at the end of this book.

Steps in Making Clinical Ethics Decisions

1. Recognize the type of problem(s).
2. Collect and clarify all medical, legal, and moral data.
3. Identify the appropriate decision maker(s).
4. Specify all options.
5. Evaluate these options.
6. Select and act on the option(s).
7. Review the case.

Step 1:
Recognize a Problem

The first step is to recognize the problem you encounter. Internal and/or external symptoms signal the presence of problems. Internal symptoms usually show themselves in changes in your behavior during clinical encounters. Awkward and uncomfortable interactions with your patients, with their family members, or with staff members, or curt responses to nurses and interns who interrupt you during your clinical workups show that your coping mechanisms are compromised. These signs signal the presence of problems. You need to clarify what they are and why they are present before proceeding with your clinical interactions.

The external signals of a problem are usually quite obvious. Patients, family members, or staff members who do not agree with your management of a case express their disagreement overtly or covertly. Overt behavior, thankfully, is rare. Nonetheless, you do encounter families and patients who show their disagreement by anger, loud and/or aggressive behavior, or by the threat of legal action. More commonly, they show disagreement in more subtle covert ways. Your patient "forgets" to take the prescribed medicine as directed or becomes stoic and sphinxlike when you ask questions. Family members badger you with phone calls. Nurses become cool and distant. You begin to feel frustrated and even a bit angry when you meet with this patient or family.

Do not ignore the presence of internal and/or external signals of a problem. You may be tempted to put on your professional face and plunge onward despite the symptoms, but the prudent course of action is to pause and sort out their cause before proceeding. Many times, the source of the problem is lack of communication. However, if the problem is confusion or conflict over obligations, you are facing a clinical predicament, a moral dilemma, or a moral quandary.

A clinical predicament is a complicated, perplexing situation from which it is difficult to disengage. A moral dilemma is a perplexing situation that requires a choice between competing obligations, many of which are equally disagreeable both to you and your patient. A moral quandary is a state of great perplexity and uncertainty caused by lack of moral knowledge. The predicament, dilemma, or quandary take on forms that range from whether you should tell a patient that he or she has a terminal illness to whether you should alter your diagnosis so that your patient will be covered financially by the HMO's business plan. Many examples of clinical problems are presented in the cases in Chapter 3 and disbursed throughout this chapter. However, the examples are not exhaustive. You will find a description of other common and not so common ethical problems in the appendix.

First Things First

A mother reacts with puzzlement and anger when the physician reports to her: "Suzy has *edema* in her belly. We are taking steps to remove it." The mother hears, "Suzy has *a demon* in her belly."

The majority of clinical predicaments are caused by ineffective communication. Many factors contribute to poor communication. Economic and managerial pressures require you to be more efficient and cost-effective. You are expected to increase the number of patients you see. Usually, the first casualty to efficiency is the amount of time you allot to explaining your diagnosis and therapeutic recommendations to patients and family members. Even the interdisciplinary nature of health care practice contributes to poor communication. Frequently, your recommendations are interpreted by and/or communicated to patients and families through nurses, fellows, resident physicians, medical students, or even by other patients and family members. Medical terminology that you use to communicate efficiently and precisely with your colleagues slips unrecognized into your conversations with patients and families. Medical language is incomprehensible jargon to most patients.

Patients and family members also unwittingly contribute to poor communication. They are anxious to learn the cause and significance of troubling symptoms. Their unfamiliarity with medical language and their fear that your diagnosis and recommendations will give them "bad news" make ineffective communication a high probability. The medical truism, "patients hear what they want to hear," contains a great deal of wisdom. Your challenge is to communicate what your patient needs to know in language, concepts, and metaphors that he or she can comprehend.

To fulfill your obligation to instruct your patients requires careful scrutiny of your ability to choose terms that avoid medical jargon and communicate effectively at your patient's level of comprehension. Fulfilling your obligation to be a teacher also requires patience. Merely asking a patient or family member "Do you have any questions about what I have told you? [Pause] No? OK! But if you think of any questions later, please have me paged" does not fulfill this obligation because most patients and family members are overwhelmed by the information you have given them and are not able to formulate questions. Also, asking your patient "Are there any words I have used that you do not understand?" is not an effective way to test your success in avoiding medical jargon. This question frequently makes a patient or family member defensive. They do not wish to appear ignorant.

To test more effectively the adequacy of your communication of diagnostic, therapeutic, and prognostic information, ask your patients what they think is causing their symptoms and whether they are willing to undergo the therapies you recommend. Pay close attention to their responses. This requires patience on your part, but patience will give you insight into how you can effectively communicate with your patients. Use of carefully prepared written, audio, and video materials can also assist in the communication process. If you discover that the predicament is not due to miscommunication, there is high probability that you are facing a moral dilemma or quandary.

Moral Dilemmas

Moral dilemmas occur when your problem is a conflict between obligations. A moral dilemma is a situation in which simultaneously you must do and not to do the same thing. Moral dilemmas occur for the following reasons: (a) competing obligations, (b) uncertainty or confusion over what obligation applies to the case, or (c) the lack of compelling reasons to follow one obligation rather than another.

The case "To Tell or Not to Tell" (p. 20) illustrates a dilemma produced by competing obligations. The ER physician, Dr. Andrews, knows he has an obligation to tell Mrs. Wilson that her husband is dead. However, through his intern, her children, Mr. and Mrs. Roberts, clearly tell him that he must not reveal Dr. Wilson's death to Mrs. Wilson when she asks about his condition. Dr. Andrews must resolve the contradiction between two compelling obligations: He must be truthful to Mrs. Wilson's direct request for information about her husband's condition, and simultaneously, he must not tell her that her husband is dead because her children warn him that revealing Dr. Wilson's death will cause psychological or physical harm to Mrs. Wilson.

A classic moral dilemma caused by conflicting duties occurs everyday in the hospital. You must decide how to manage the pain of a dying patient. Mrs. Oma is in great pain. She is a terminally ill 89-year-old woman whose years of smoking have brought her to end-stage lung cancer. Her pain is managed only by increasing the frequency and amount of her morphine. You know that morphine has two effects: It controls Mrs. Oma's pain, but it also suppresses her diminishing lung function. You have tried other pain control methods but with no success. Increasing the morphine does relieve her pain but also shortens her life. Simultaneously, you must reduce Mrs. Oma's pain and not harm her. The same action (giving morphine) produces both desirable and undesirable results. You must and must not do the same thing.

The case "To Treat or Not to Treat"(p. 22) is another example of a dilemma caused by competing obligations. Dr. Bronski is convinced that he has an obligation to transfuse Mr. Jove because a blood transfusion is medically indicated to give him a chance to survive. However, Mr. Jove and his family have different moral perceptions. Because of their religion, they believe a blood transfusion carries severe negative religious and social consequences. They feel strongly that they have an obligation to thwart Dr. Bronski's attempts to get them to agree to blood transfusion.

Although many moral dilemmas are caused by competing obligations, they are also caused by moral uncertainty or confusion over obligations. In the case of "The Noble Volunteer" (p. 34), Mrs. Alton is willing to sacrifice the use of her nondominant thumb to assist medical researchers in their search for a cure to Parkinson's disease. The resident physician is uncertain whether he can responsibly accept Mrs. Alton's offer to serve as a control in the experiment. He knows her offer will result in irreversible injury to her thumb, but Mrs. Alton's offer also may provide valuable information for the treatment of future Parkinson's patients. The resident's understanding of what is morally acceptable and unacceptable is unclear.

Finally, moral dilemmas occur when there is a lack of compelling reasons to support one obligation rather than another. Dr. Bronski ("To Treat or Not to Treat?" p. 22) faces a dilemma because the strong reason supporting blood transfusion for a trauma patient is opposed by an equally strong argument to honor Mr. Jove's wishes. Nurses, residents, and technicians in Dr. Bronski's intensive care unit support opposite actions. The split in his staff members and the family's unanimous support of Mr. Jove's rejection of blood put Dr.

Bronski at risk no matter what he decides to do. Dr. Bronski is experiencing the stress of trying to reach a decision that is professionally, legally, and culturally acceptable when the medical profession and society have not definitively decided which position's arguments are more compelling.

Moral Quandary

You are in a moral quandary when you find yourself in an unprecedented situation. To make a choice in a moral quandary, you must step into uncharted areas and take the risk of social, professional, and legal disapproval or condemnation. Fortunately, moral quandaries rarely occur in clinical practice. However, when new medical technology becomes available or research breakthroughs occur, their implications for clinical practice can produce moral quandaries. For example, the success of heart, liver, and pancreas transplantation furthered by the development of antirejection drugs, such as cyclosporin, create unprecedented dilemmas for the clinician. These quandaries concern procurement of organs, selection of candidates, distribution of organs, and even interspecies transplantation. Perhaps the most dramatic of these moral quandaries is xenograph transplantation. When the cardiac surgeon decided to replace an infant girl's severely genetically deformed heart with a baboon's heart, he had no direct moral precedent to justify his decision. He probably used a traditional medical rule "he must save the life of his patient" to justify his decision to proceed. He saw xenograph as the only procedure available to him to save the infant girl. However, a contemporary comment describes the xenograph transplant as a suspect experiment teetering on the edge of the unethical. Today, the unlocking of the secrets of the human genome and the role of DNA in the etiology of disease raise moral quandaries about the clinical use of this knowledge as well as the disclosure of genetic information about individual patients for insurance underwriting, employment, and so on.

Step 2:
Collect and Clarify Data

The aphorism "The beginning of prescription is description" summarizes the next step in clinical ethics decision making. As noted above, frequently, the cause of a clinical predicament can be traced to ineffective communication, a misunderstanding of language, law, factual data, or the meaning or applicability of moral knowledge.

Medical Data

When there is ambiguity or confusion over the thoroughness, reliability, and validity of diagnostic tests or over the interpretation of such tests, fresh review of the data is required.

> Mr. Willy, a 65-year-old retired steelworker, is hospitalized with symptoms of nausea, some vague left arm weakness, and dizziness. Dr. Elmer, the admitting physician, notes that Mr. Willy's medical history is remarkable for a transient ischemic accident (TIA) six years ago that left him with no deficits. Suspicion that another neurological event is occurring prompts Dr. Elmer to order blood thinners to reduce the chances of neurological damage and to order extensive radiographic tests. All test results are ambiguous and the symptoms continue. Dr. Elmer discusses the problem with Mr. Willy: "We may need to go in to see if we can find what is causing your symptoms." Mr. Willy agrees to have a neurosurgeon, Dr. Eberly, examine him. Mr. Willy is apprehensive about surgery but is adamant that Dr. Elmer take steps to find the cause or causes of his symptoms.
>
> The next morning, Dr. Smith, Dr. Eberly's fellow, performs a complete history and physical in preparation for Dr. Eberly's visit. During the physical examination, Dr. Smith discovers a large buildup of wax in Mr. Willy's ear canals. He asks Mr. Willy whether anyone had examined his ears while he was in the hospital. Mr. Willy says, "No. I don't remember anyone sticking that thing in my ears."
>
> Dr. Smith flushes out the wax. By midmorning, Mr. Willy's symptoms are greatly diminished. Further neurological examination and observation confirm that the symptoms very probably were caused by the wax buildup in Mr. Willy's ears.

Mr. Willy's case shows the importance of gathering all medical data and challenging assumptions. Furthermore, thoroughness in examination and management contributes to establishing an empirical and ethical baseline for therapeutic decisions. Second opinions and consultations are necessary for thoroughness. Even when consultations and second opinions produce conflicting diagnoses and/or therapeutic recommendations, they raise important questions that must be clarified before decisions are made.

Moral and Legal Information

Gathering and clarifying moral and legal information are as critical to avoiding and resolving clinical predicaments as gathering and clarifying medical data. Frequently, legal information is found in hospital policy and procedure manuals. Nonetheless, legal information is best gathered and clarified by consultation with hospital legal counsel before a crisis occurs. Everyone brings moral knowledge to the clinical workup. You, your patients, and their family members bring expectations about the right and wrong way to interact with each other. These expectations range from questions of etiquette (do not address your doctor, or patient, by first name) to moral ideas of right and wrong behavior (the doctors must keep personal information confidential; patients must tell the doctor the truth about their symptoms). Ironically, you and your patients' moral expectations contribute to or even cause predicaments or dilemmas to occur.

Moral Rules

You and your patients bring two types of moral knowledge to the clinical meeting. The first is a loose collection of rules of conduct that express obligations in direct clear language. These rules are often aphorisms ("honesty is the best policy") or claims of a "right" to take action or to be left undisturbed ("I have a right to choose my doctor." "The patient has a right to die." "As a doctor, I have a right to accept or not accept a patient.") or codes of conduct such as the Ten Commandments (Thou shall . . .; Thou shall not . . .).

Codes of medical ethics are part of the medical tradition. Written codes of medical ethics are very important resources. However, the unwritten rules of conduct acquired from your mentors are more effective in your development of practical ways to respond to problems. For example, one of the most powerful unwritten medical rules is, "You must save your patient's life." This rule directs physicians' decisions about initiating and continuing life-sustaining and life-supporting technology. These decisions are made without question and, at times, without the patient's or family's knowledge or approval.

In the United States, many rules of conduct are legal "rights." A right is a claim that a person is empowered to do something (aka, a positive right: I have a right to make my own decisions about therapy) or that he or she is to be undisturbed (aka, a negative right: I have the right to privacy). The basis for these rights is found in (a) law—the government gives rights to its citizens through passing laws and judicial decisions (e.g., only physicians have the right to pre-scribe controlled substances); (b) a privilege granted to certain persons (e.g., your congressperson has the privilege of mailing his or her correspondence without paying postage); or (c) tradition (e.g., in this city, physicians are not ticketed for traffic violations). The use of the word *right* assumes that there is a privilege, law, or judicial ruling that empowers you in a certain way. It can also mean that your cultural and/or professional tradition has developed rules of conduct that give you a "right" to act in a certain way.

However, rules of conduct have limitations. They are specific and impera-tive. They are very much like laws. Rules of conduct give instructions, and you are expected to follow them or face the consequences. Rules, like laws, do not allow for discussion. They direct your action and serve as judges of your guilt or innocence. For example, after you are stopped by a policeman who sees you merely slow down at a stop sign, you protest, "But Officer, there was no traffic in any direction when I coasted through the stop sign. I rushed through because I am late for a job interview." The policeman shows no sympathy as he takes your license and insurance card. "Sorry! I am writing you a ticket. Please sign here. Your signature does not mean you admit you are guilty. Your guilt and penalty will be decided by the traffic court judge."

Rules of conduct do not anticipate all circumstances and conditions. You quickly learn in your clinical rotations that you must "call a code when your patient has a cardiac arrest." The rule to call a code does not have nuances built into it because nuances would make the rule cumbersome and difficult to fol-low. Nevertheless, if you do not call the resuscitation team and your patient suffers injury or death, you will be expected to demonstrate cogent reasons for not following the rule. By relying on the next type of moral knowledge, moral value, you may be able to justify why you did not follow the rule to call a code.

Moral Values

The second type of moral knowledge that you and your patients bring to the clinical encounter is moral values. Unlike rules of conduct, moral values are abstract directions rather than concrete orders. Moral values are generalized expectations about the relationships between persons and between persons and institutions. You expect to be treated fairly and respectfully by your medical school instructors (the values of justice and respect for persons); you expect a secure campus environment so that no harm comes to you or your colleagues (the value of life); you want the opportunity to make your own choices (the value of individual freedom). Because moral values are abstract, they do not specify what action, rule, or policy will provide safety, give freedom, and be fair in different circumstances. Much like the Supreme Court justice's comment about the definition of obscenity ("I know it when I see it"), moral values are recognized by their presence or, more often, by their absence.

Moral values are very useful in resolving moral dilemmas and quandaries. When you must act in circumstances that require more than mere adherence to a rule of conduct, moral values give direction for finding a solution. For example, the rule that requires you to call a code when your patient has a cardiac arrest is based on the assumption that your patient's life is important (value of life) and that he or she wants to be resuscitated (value of personal freedom). If your patient is in end-stage disease with multiple organ failure, has an advanced directive for health care decisions that explicitly rejects resuscitation under these circumstances, and has a family that supports the advanced directive, cardiac resuscitation would be inappropriate because it would disregard the values of respect for a person's free choice, his or her understanding of a meaningful life, and the social value of economic fairness.

Step 3:
Identify the Decision Makers

Mr. Shawon Jamal is a 55-year-old lawyer admitted to University Hospital five days ago because of a suspected heart attack. His symptoms were successfully treated. After being stabilized, he underwent a diagnostic angiogram. He is now resting comfortably in his hospital room waiting for a visit from his cardiologist, Dr. Blumenthal. Dr. Blumenthal is a burly gray-haired man who has been in practice for 30 years. He is widely respected in the medical community as an astute diagnostician and for remaining at the cutting edge of cardiology. A large smile lights up Dr. Blumenthal's face as he walks into Mr. Jamal's hospital room.

He greets Mr. Jamal with a firm handshake. "Well, you had a rough time, but now we have some answers. You did have a heart attack. The good news is you suffered only minor muscle damage to your heart. The bad news is your angiogram shows 80% to 90% blockage in two of your cardiac arteries. You are a prime candidate for another heart attack. This leaves us with no choice. I have scheduled you for bypass surgery next week."

Dr. Blumenthal is surprised by Mr. Jamal's refusal to undergo surgery. "I don't want surgery. I will try diet, exercise, and drugs instead of surgery."

Dr. Blumenthal smoothly responds: "Well, Mr. Jamal, I understand your concern about surgery, but you don't need to decide now. Think it over. I will be back this afternoon to discuss this with you again." He pauses and continues: "I really recommend surgery for you. You have a full life ahead of you. You do want to see your grandchildren grow up. Surgery will give you the chance."

As Dr. Blumenthal walks down the corridor to his next patient's room, he stops and tells his residents and medical students, "Mr. Jamal is a patient who thinks he knows more than the doctor. I've faced them before, but I must admit rejection of my advice always makes my blood boil. You need to learn to control your feelings when talking with your patients. You always must act in their best interest and not give them a reason to lose confidence in you. Even though Mr. Jamal is a lawyer, his next angina attack will change his mind."

Dr. Blumenthal's feelings of anger are understandable. Making clinical decisions requires competence, knowledge, experience, and authority. His education, training, and years of experience support his analysis and decision to schedule Mr. Jamal for bypass surgery. The decision to schedule bypass surgery is backed by solid medical reasons and is motivated by Dr. Blumenthal's desire to choose what is in Mr. Jamal's "best interest." However, despite his altruistic motivation, Dr. Blumenthal neglected to discuss the need for surgery with Mr. Jamal before scheduling it, and he did not ask Mr. Jamal's reasons for rejecting surgery. Furthermore, Dr. Blumenthal only gives lip service to Mr. Jamal's being the decision maker. ". . . his next angina attack will change his mind."

Learning the role and responsibilities of being a decision maker is embedded in your medical curricula. The deference given to you by the lay public reinforces that role. Naturally, your education and experience create the assumption that you, as physician, should make clinical decisions in your patient's best interest. There is no doubt that you experience the heavy burdens of making clinical choices. The wrong diagnosis or the choice of an ineffective or harmful therapy exposes you to professional and legal sanctions. However, it is presumptuous for you to make decisions for your patients without understanding their personal aspirations, goals, and values.

The question of who is the appropriate decision maker frequently arises in the following situations:

- End-of-life decisions
- Pediatric care (especially in cases in which instituting or withdrawing life support decisions must be made)
- Care of adolescents (when is an adolescent independent from parents in medical decisions?)
- Care of the mentally and emotionally challenged patient (see the case of Ms. Adams, "To Operate or Not to Operate?" p. 29).

Many of the cases presented in Chapter 3 illustrate the tug-of-war that occurs when a patient or family desires one course of action and the physician another. A classic example is the case of Mrs. Mancini ("A Family Divided," p. 24) in which the question is whether to escalate or withhold life support therapy. The family members have different opinions. Some insist that "everything must be done." Some want to stop therapy. Others are ambivalent. Mrs. Mancini's physician, Dr. Aurelio, feels that she has an obligation to discontinue what she considers a futile therapy. Continuing to treat Mrs. Mancini would seriously violate Dr. Aurelio's conscience even though some family members insist she must continue. Who is empowered to decide when there is disagreement?

The rule of conduct that identifies the appropriate decision maker is this: The person most directly affected by the decision is the appropriate decision maker. The competent, well-informed patient is the appropriate decision maker. However, Mrs. Mancini is not a competent patient. Unfortunately, she did not prepare a legal document, an advanced directive, that expresses her end-of-life wishes and/or appoints someone to make these decisions for her. Because the family is divided and Dr. Aurelio feels she should not escalate therapy, a conflict over who is the decision maker occurs. When the attempt to identify the appropriate decision maker reaches an impasse, each medical institution should have in place services, policies, or procedures that assist resolution of the impasse. When all attempts fail to resolve an impasse, the "court of last appeal" is the judicial system. Suggestions about institutional policies and procedures are discussed in Chapter 6.

Open discussion with your patients about end-of-life decisions will reduce the possibility of conflicts over who is the decision maker. Early in your clinical relationship, ask whether your patients have thought about their lifelong goals and aspirations and discussed their end-of-life wishes with their loved ones and/or lawyers. Ask if there is anyone they have appointed as decision maker for them in the event they become incompetent to make medical decisions. Find out whether they have prepared advanced directives.

Every state in the United States has legislation usually described as "advance directives" to address the question of who has the right to make medical decisions when the patient is incapacitated. The title indicates that the law's intention is to protect patients' rights to *give directions* for medical decision making *in advance* of circumstances in which they will not be competent to make medical decisions. Through these directives, patients empower person(s) with the authority and obligation to make medical decisions for them when they are incapable of doing so. There are two forms of advance directives: a living will and a durable power of attorney for health care choices. Definitions of these advance directives are in the glossary at the end of the book.

Some of the most distressing conflicts over identifying decision makers occur in pediatric cases. Parents have the authority and obligation to make medical decisions for their underage children. Nonetheless, pediatricians and other medical personnel usually have very strong feelings about their own obligations to protect children from harm, especially when their medical judgment about therapy conflicts with parents' judgment. In most cases, conflict over the questions of therapy (such as nontraditional cancer therapy) requires consultation, negotiation, and in some cases, judicial intervention.

Adolescent patients as well as intellectually and physically challenged patients, raise even more thorny questions about competency. Again, the physician's obligation to protect patients and to act in their best interest may conflict with parents and guardians' judgment about what in fact will protect their children. These conflicts can result in tugs-of-war over identifying the appropriate decision maker.

In conclusion, to avoid struggles over who has the authority and obligation to make medical decisions, prepare your patients for these decisions by encouraging them to prepare advance directives. When you face a potential conflict with a patient or family, create an environment in which all parties contribute information and their unique perspectives to the task of decision making. You contribute the medical data and the prognosis. Your patient and their family members contribute personal life goals and thoughts about circumstances in which they may wish to limit or stop therapy. Ideally, a consensus can be reached among all parties to proceed along a course set by all. When pains are taken to create this environment of cooperation, the question of who is the appropriate decision maker rarely arises. All parties participate in the decision. No party is arbitrarily excluded.

Step 4:
Specify All Options

The Reverend Reynolds's wife (p. 35) places doctors in a serious predicament. Her strong religious belief thwarts all attempts to persuade her to agree to the removal of ventilator and dialysis support from her brain-dead husband. She is adamant in her belief that he will recover. His physicians feel that any further attempts to change her mind will be fruitless and will only alienate her. The case is quickly turning into a confrontation of beliefs and a battle of wills.

The physicians feel angry and frustrated. They are angry because Mrs. Reynolds cannot or will not see the reasonableness of the doctors' recommendations. They are frustrated because they are unable to discontinue life support. Anger and frustration siphon off the intellectual and creative energy necessary to identify options.

Dr. Simon, the head of critical care medicine, calls a meeting to devise a strategy to solve the problem. In attendance are the critical care physicians and nurses in charge of Pastor Reynolds's care, the hospital's ethicist, chaplain, attorney, and community relations director. Dr. Simon outlines the obvious options of continuing the current level of life support or stopping all life support despite Mrs. Reynolds's objections. The group rejects both options. Continuing life support for a clinically diagnosed brain-dead patient is an unacceptable use of financial, physical, and personnel resources. But a unilateral decision to discontinue life support is a callous disregard for Mrs. Reynolds's faith and her authority to act as Reverend Reynolds's surrogate decision maker. Furthermore, unilateral stopping of life support could result in bad publicity and possible legal action against the physicians and hospital. The impasse is deep. The doctors report that Mrs. Reynolds rejects all reasonable explanations for discontinuing life support. She firmly believes that God will "resurrect" her husband and she knows that Pastor Reynolds would not allow any cessation of life support. "He would never give up hope and trust in God."

Dr. Simon introduces the option of "damage control." Can the hospital manage the negative fallout of either disregarding Mrs. Reynolds's wishes or following her wishes? The attorney outlines the pertinent state laws and indicates how a local jury would probably react to the hospital's argument that stopping life support despite Mrs. Reynolds's wishes is medically and legally defensible. The chaplain describes in detail the theological basis for Mrs. Reynolds's belief and her frustrating attempt to persuade Mrs. Reynolds that her religion does not require continued life support in these circumstances.

The conference room falls silent. No one seems willing to accept the "damage control" option to settle the impasse. Then the ethicist asks, "Can we cut our losses by a compromise solution?" When asked to expand on his comment the ethicist responds: "Can the physicians accept part of what Mrs. Reynolds wants and ask her to accept part of what the physicians want?" The conference room buzzes with conversations. Physicians and nurses offer a compromise. "We can agree to continue life support at the present level but draw the line at resuscitation. The history of these cases shows that cardiac and/or pulmonary arrest will occur. Although a technically successful resuscitation is possible in these circumstances, the resuscitation obviously will not change the diagnosis of brain death." The chaplain suggests, "We ask Mrs. Reynolds to trust her God to give a signal that He is calling Pastor Reynolds to his eternal reward rather than using the doctors to bring him back to his flock. The most obvious signal would be God's stopping his heart." The plan is accepted and put into motion. Mrs. Reynolds agrees to the plan. Pastor Reynolds's heart stops two days later, and no resuscitation attempts are made.

Enlist the minds and imaginations of persons not directly involved in a clinical case and encourage an open discussion of all possible options. Frequently, this results in the discovery of options that are not obvious to the participants in the dispute.

Step 5:
Evaluate Options

After you identify all the options to resolve a predicament, dilemma, or quandary, evaluate the options. This task requires comparing the options to the moral knowledge and legal precedents that apply to the case. Obviously, legal perspective is best obtained by consulting with your hospital attorneys. It is important to approach attorneys with well-defined questions about the legal implications of your predicament and to be clear that you are seeking legal opinion and not asking the attorney to solve the case for you. The burden of decision is yours.

Before you approach legal counsel for advice, review the moral rules of conduct and moral values that apply to your case to clarify your questions. The review process will also specify questions about the legal implications for your proposed course of action that can be presented to your hospital attorney. Although the following moral values and rules of conduct are not exhaustive, I have found them useful in finding options to resolve the most common clinical ethics problems. Most predicaments and dilemmas involve questions of life, autonomy (freedom), or justice.

Life

Life is both a biological and moral concept. Biologically, "life" describes an organism's ability to function and grow to maturity. Absence of function and cessation of growth indicate the opposite of life, death. Life as a moral value is expressed in the pithy statement: "If you do not have life you have nothing." Life is valued, fostered, and preserved by persons because life is the basis for all their interpersonal and human activities that range from reproduction to production of products, relationships, art, and knowledge.

The moral value of life is the basis for your duty to preserve life. But "The devil is in the details." Do you have a duty to preserve the life of this patient? Must you continue to sustain the life of a terminally ill patient for whom no therapy is available? The following list of conditions either intensify or weaken your duty to preserve the life of a patient.

- Intensifying conditions
    - A life-threatening or life diminishing condition
    - Presence of effective medical treatment
    - Capacity or potential for establishing interpersonal relationships
    - Capacity for making autonomous decisions

- Weakening conditions
    - Diagnosis of end-stage illness
    - Ineffective medical interventions

– Diminished or absent ability to maintain interpersonal relationships
– Diminished or absent capacity to decide

Several rules of conduct flow from the value to preserve and foster your patients' lives. These rules of conduct are moral standards for care of your patients.

Traditionally, these rules of conduct are expressed as "Do not harm your patient" and "Act in your patient's best interest." Again, "The devil is in the details." Exactly which actions will harm and which will benefit your patient? Although answers to these perplexing questions can be found only in the context of a specific case, there is a practice guideline that requires you to search for therapies that will balance positive and negative results of your therapeutic decision.

The reality of clinical decision making is that you rarely perform a procedure or prescribe a drug that does not carry with it the potential for negative side effects. Even suturing a laceration and giving antibiotics to battle infection carries the negative side effects of a scar and the possible allergic reaction to the antibiotic. The guiding principle here is to balance the positive and negative results of choosing a therapy for your patient.

Your training and continuing education give you the information, skill, and experience to weigh the medical benefits and harms of any therapy. The danger is that you will judge benefit and harm to your patient solely in medical terms. Benefit and harm, like beauty, are in the eye of the beholder. In other words, you and the patient may place different values on the options. Be sure that you understand the way your patient perceives benefits and harms. Your patient's perception of what is good for him or her and what is bad for him or her is critical to the selection of therapies.

Dr. Blumenthal (p. 55) is surprised by Mr. Jamal's decision to reject cardiac bypass as a therapeutic option. The decision makes no sense to Dr. Blumenthal because the risks of the cardiac surgery are so low and the benefits to Mr. Jamal so great. Dr. Blumenthal is correct, medically speaking. Cardiac surgery is indicated medically for Mr. Jamal who is otherwise healthy and very intelligent. However, Dr. Blumenthal did not discuss surgery with Mr. Jamal before he scheduled surgery, and he did not invite Mr. Jamal to explain his concerns about cardiothoracic surgery. Because Mr. Jamal is a lawyer, he may be automatically reacting negatively to Dr. Blumenthal's announcement. Lawyers are very sensitive to protecting the rights of their clients. Mr. Jamal may interpret Dr. Blumenthal's scheduling surgery without his approval as a violation of his patient rights. Another possibility is that although Mr. Jamal is well educated, he may have incorrect information about cardiac surgery or he may have other personal and professional priorities that prompt him to reject surgery. If Dr. Blumenthal asks Mr. Jamal why he chooses a regimen of diet, exercise, and drugs over surgery, he might learn that Mr. Jamal vicariously experienced his elder brother's very difficult bypass surgery 10 years ago and his brother's long (1 year) convalescence before returning to his work. That his brother was older, sicker, and did not have the advantage of current surgical advancements is important information for Mr. Jamal to consider and perhaps reassess his judgment about surgery. Or Dr. Blumenthal might learn that Mr. Jamal is currently engaged in a delicate and intricate legal case that may lead to significant professional and financial gain for him and his family. He may want to reduce to a minimum the delay in returning to preparing the briefs for this case. In any scenario, Dr. Blumenthal needs information about how Mr. Jamal perceives risk and benefit. This information will provide grounds for further discussion and a mutually agreeable course of action.

Autonomy

The moral value of autonomy is the expectation that persons should make their own decisions without coercion or manipulation. A free person chooses to act in ways that are consistent with the plan he or she has developed to reach personally defined goals. An autonomous person is independent, self-reliant, and has the capacity to make decisions.

The value of personal freedom is the basis for your duty to respect your patients' choices even when their choices put them at risk or seem to be foolish or unreasonable to you. However, your duty to respect your patient's decisions is not an absolute duty. There are conditions that either reduce your duty or place the burden of decision making on you and/or your patient's surrogate decision makers. These conditions are the following:

- Diminished understanding
- Diminished capacity to make choices
- High dependency on others

When these conditions are present, the obligation to protect your patient is stronger than the obligation to respect his or her choices.

Questions of respecting persons and their choices arise both in dramatic and humdrum circumstances. An example of the dramatic clash between personal autonomies is seen in the case "Please Help Me!" (p. 19). The case raises

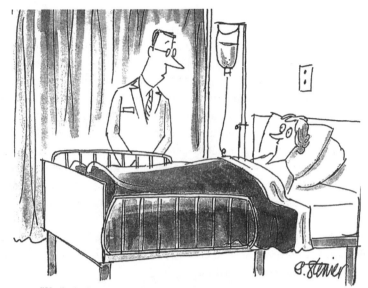

"Medical ethics do not allow me to assist in your death. I am, however,
permitted to keep you miserable as long as possible."

a very delicate question about personal freedom and the duty to protect. Mrs.
Olson begs Dr. Byrn to give her an overdose of morphine because she cannot
tolerate the pain of her end-stage cancer. His response is, "I cannot do that.
This will make you comfortable." Dr. Byrn and Mrs. Olson are autonomous
persons. Each has their own vision of what they wish to be and to accomplish.
Their freedoms clash. Dr. Byrn wants to finish his residency without con-
troversy, and he wishes to avoid harming Mrs. Olson. Mrs. Olson wants to die
on her own terms, but the drugs that will bring her death are under Dr. Byrn's
control.

The questions that plague Dr. Byrn are whether he has a duty to respect Mrs.
Olson's request: Does her disease diminish her capacity to decide? How will
his colleagues and mentors judge him if he overdoses her or if he ignores her
request? A safe course to follow is to obtain a professional opinion about Mrs.
Olson's capacity to decide and to arrange for religious and psychological support. Unless these tactics demonstrate that she is incapacitated, Dr. Byrn still
faces the choice of respecting or ignoring her wishes. The burden of decision
is his.

Medical practice and social policy do not support either euthanasia or
assisted suicide. However, the argument that "the duty to respect a competent

patient's wishes overrides the duty to prevent harm" has growing support mainly because the advancement of medical technology has created a "Frankenstein" effect: Medical techniques sustain life in persons who are tortured by the awareness of dying in painful and demeaning circumstances.

Questions of autonomy also occur in the humdrum daily activities of a doctor's practice. The simple act of writing a prescription and giving instructions for taking the prescription assumes that your patient agrees to follow your advice. You are expected to inform the patient about her illness, the therapy that should effectively control or cure her illness, the possible side effects of the drugs you are prescribing, and the prognosis. The information is intended to allow your patient to willingly consent to follow the therapy you have outlined. You expect your patient to give you an informed consent.

Although informed consent is a phrase normally used to describe a patient's agreement to participate in medical research, the phrase also describes a patient's agreement to undergo diagnostic and therapeutic procedures. The concept of informed consent rests on the value of autonomy. When a senior physician asks you to "get informed consent" or "to consent the patient," your obligation is to use comprehensible language to explain the therapy. Be certain that the patient understands. Respect the patient's freedom to accept or reject the therapy. Patient consent must be informed and voluntary. The challenge is to choose verbal and body language that clearly gives information and avoids any manipulation. Patients may ask you, "What would you do?" To respond, "It is your decision" is not acceptable. The patient may be seeking support for his or her choice or a forum to address fears or questions. Inquire, "Why do you want my opinion?" This inquiry could reveal the patient's motivation for asking you and also provide an opportunity for addressing the patient's questions or fears.

Justice

Christine is a third-year medical student assigned to Dr. Sylvia Phillips, the head of Pediatrics. Christine is convinced that using small gifts of candy as a reward to young children after they have been examined will give children a positive impression of doctors that will last them through their adult life. She carries a supply of sugarless lollipops in her white coat.

Mrs. Oliver brings her four-year-old twins into the examining room. Charlie is fine, but Jack has a slight fever and earache. Dr. Phillips asks Mrs. Oliver whether she will allow Christine, a medical student, to examine Jack's ears. Mrs. Oliver agrees and holds Jack while Christine examines his ears and gives him a brief physical examination. Although Jack is apprehensive about Christine's putting the otoscope into his ear, he does not resist because Christine's calming voice and smooth manner reassure him. When she finishes Christine reaches into her pocket and produces a lollipop for Jack, saying, "You are a good patient, Jack. Here's your reward." To her amazement, Charlie, who had been quietly watching and sucking his thumb, bursts into tears and cries out, "That's not fair! I want a lolly too. I've been a good boy!" Dr. Phillips quickly picks up Charlie and says, "Well, Charlie, if you let me examine your ears I will give you a lollipop." This quiets Charlie. He bravely holds up his head and allows Dr. Phillips to insert the otoscope into his ears. Charlie and Jack leave the examination room happily licking their lollipops.

Charlie's outburst is understandable. Children are acutely aware of inequality and offer loud, if inarticulate, commentaries about inequality, usually by crying out, "That's not fair!" Charlie's loud complaint expresses his awareness that he has been treated differently than Jack; he feels he has been discriminated against even though he has no idea of the meaning of discrimination. Charlie thinks he also deserves a lollipop because he "has been good" too. He sat quietly sucking his thumb while his mother held Jack.

The best way to understand the moral value of justice is to understand the idea of "deserving something." Justice is present when a person receives what he or she deserves or can legitimately claim. Charlie does not deserve a lollipop because he did not undergo the ear examination. Nonetheless, Charlie wants a lollipop. His sense of unfairness, unequal treatment, sparks his crying. Dr. Phillips wisely subjects Charlie to the same examination so that there is, in fact, equality between Jack and Charlie's claims and rewards. Both allow their ears to be examined with the otoscope, and both claim their reward.

The moral value of justice concerns the distribution of benefits and burdens. The most troubling questions concern the distribution of benefits when there are limited benefits and competing claims for these benefits. These questions go beyond the scope of this book. Nonetheless, you face changes in social policy concerning reimbursements to you and the availability of economic resources for your patients' medical expenses. Practicing medicine in the 21st century brings with it the responsibility to become a participant, at least on the local level, in the political and economic discussions about distribution of medical services and reimbursement. You have the knowledge and the experience to bring reality to these discussions.

Step 6:
Select an Option and Act

The practical guideline for selecting an option is to choose the option that best answers the medical and moral questions raised by the case. Usually, this is achieved by some form of compromise in which the parties accept a limited solution. The case of the Reverend Reynolds (pp. 35 and 59-60) illustrates a compromise solution to what seems to be an irreconcilable difference of opinion. The reason the compromise is accepted by all parties in the Reynolds case is that both groups permit limits to their own perceived obligations. Mrs. Reynolds agrees to a limitation of therapy; the physicians agree to continue life support therapy to a certain point.

Many times, the compromise solution can be achieved only if persons, places, and procedures are changed. This can be facilitated by the introduction of neutral leaders (e.g., an ethics consultant or ethics committee) to guide the discussion.

Meetings are held in a conference room removed from the clinical environment. The meeting's ground rules encourage open discussion of options and suggestions rather than merely the communication of information and expectation of decisions. These changes create an environment of cooperation rather than confrontation that leads to solutions for perplexing predicaments and dilemmas.

You also have an ethical obligation regarding the way you fulfill your responsibilities.

Mrs. Winston, the 36-year-old wife of an electrical company lineman, is escorted by the state police to a hospital ER because her husband has been in a serious accident. He and his crew were clearing away debris from the recent devastating snow and ice storm. All she knows is that while removing limbs and trees from the electrical lines, her husband was struck without warning by an "exploding" tree. She knows he is alive but does not know anything further about his condition.

Mrs. Winston is nervously pacing in the crowded ER waiting room. Inside the ER, doctors and nurses work feverishly to stabilize the seriously injured Mr. Winston. He was struck in the back and sustained injuries to his spine. The prognosis does not look good. When the X rays are returned, the facts are clear. A nurse reports that Mrs. Winston is in the waiting room, anxiously wanting information.

Mrs. Winston looks up when a physician dressed in scrubs calls her name. The young doctor is a stranger to her. He walks over and announces, "Your husband's spine is badly injured. His C-5 vertebra is crushed. And the C-4 is flipped over on top of the C-5. Mr. Winston is a quadriplegic and he will be for the rest of his life." Without another word, the doctor turns away and walks through the swinging doors into the ER.

The ER physician fulfills his duty to inform Mrs. Winston. She has a "right to know," and he has the duty, no matter how distasteful, to tell her. He reveals the diagnosis and prognosis frankly and accurately. However, his technique is brusque and insensitive. He does not take Mrs. Winston to a quiet private place; he gives the information in the middle of a crowded waiting room. No arrangements are made for a social worker, chaplain, or grief counselor to provide support for Mrs. Winston after she hears the grim news. The doctor does not wait for Mrs. Winston's response. He walks away, presumably to tend to other patients in the ER. This incident illustrates that in addition to being responsible to fulfill duties, you are also responsible for the way you choose to fulfill those duties.

Step 7:
Review the Case

The final step in the ethics decision-making model is to follow up each case after it is completed. I recommend a systematic review of the handling of each case for two reasons. First, the review will enable you to improve your ethics decision-making abilities by indicating strengths and weaknesses in the process; second, the review will also create a "file" of experiences that you can access when the next case arises. Although each clinical case is unique, usually there are similarities that allow you to use previous experiences to guide your approach to the new case. Your previous experiences filter the data from the new case and emphasize where the new case is unique and where it is similar or identical to previous cases.

Review of each case contributes both to the store of moral knowledge concerning the intricacies of each case and to the usefulness of various procedures, such as information-gathering techniques and family versus staff conferences. The review can take the form of a meeting in which participants offer their assessment of the overall management of the case, the process of ethics decision making, and the outcomes. A well-prepared paper or electronic interview can also serve as a forum for case review. Nurses' perceptions are especially invaluable to learn how effectively and sensitively the case has been handled. The follow-up should, if at all possible and where appropriate, include all the participants, medical staff, patients, and family members. The follow-up can be accomplished by telephone or by a mailed interview form that invites participants to share their perceptions of the way decisions were handled as well as the outcomes of the case.

5 How Do I Do It?

Taking the Role of Decision Maker

This chapter applies the ethics decision-making model to clinical stories, also know as clinical cases. Each clinical story is presented with the circumstances that give each its unique flavor and challenge. The chapter is designed so that you are the protagonist in each story. As you read the story, formulate your decision and the reasons for your choice. After each case, a detailed analysis is presented and recommended actions are outlined.

Your First Patient

Time: The present
Place: A large teaching hospital affiliated with a medical school
Cast of characters:

> **Peter Brown, M.D.,** a cardiologist and a professor of medicine
> **Mrs. Edith Glotz,** a patient
> **Jeanne Sims,** a fourth-year medical student **to be played by YOU**

> Dr. Brown tells you: "Sims, you are ready to solo. Take a history from our new admission in Room 314. When you finish her history, page me and I will help you examine her." He hands you the patient's chart and turns to answer a nurse's question about another patient.

Dr. Brown's confidence in you makes you feel good. Although he is nearing retirement, he still has the reputation of being a very demanding clinical instructor, but you also feel anxious. You hope you do not make mistakes. You read the admitting doctor's notes and the nurse practitioners' comments. Mrs. Edith Glotz is a 73-year-old grandmother whose son brought her to the local ER at the community hospital because she experienced difficulty breathing, nausea, and chest pain. An electrocardiogram supports the ER doctor's suspicion that Mrs. Glotz has had a heart attack. Her son insisted that she be transferred to University Hospital for treatment. The ER doctor made the arrangements for her admission to University Hospital's cardiology unit.

Several questions run through your head as you walk to her room. "How should I introduce myself? I am a medical student. Should I call myself *Dr. Sims?*" Although you have watched a number of your seniors do "H&P's" (patient histories and physical examinations), you are uncertain about how you should begin the interview. Some doctors are very formal. They introduce themselves as "Dr."; some do not use titles and merely say, "I am Jean Sims, your doctor"; some do not introduce themselves to the patient but simply ask the patient questions about his or her past medical history. Some address patients by their first names; others always say Mrs., Mr., or Ms. Some use colloquial or slang expressions, such as "Hi, Buddy" or "Hello Dear." Still others do not address their patients at all but merely perform the H&P with a minimum of conversation. What should you do?

Application of the six steps of ethics decision making described in the previous chapter will help you decide how to start your first solo history taking:

- Recognize the type of problem(s).
- Collect and clarify all medical, legal, and moral data.
- Identify the appropriate decision maker(s).
- Specify all options.
- Evaluate these options.
- Select and act on the option(s).
- Review the case.

Analysis

1. Recognize the ethical moment. Be quick to perceive whenever you are hearing or thinking the words "*should* I . . . ?" "*ought* I . . . ?" "*must* I . . . ?" If you are hearing or thinking these words, an ethical question is very likely waiting for you. The two questions in this case (how *should* I introduce myself? How *should* I address Mrs. Glotz?) appear, on the surface, to be questions of etiquette and "bedside manners." But in fact, both raise ethical issues.

How you should introduce yourself raises the question of whether you may use a "white lie," a deception, to gain Mrs. Glotz's confidence and cooperation. Furthermore, the way you choose to address Mrs. Glotz (by title, first name, or not at all) opens or closes the door to shared confidences and compliance. The way you introduce yourself and address your patient can harm or help your patient. These questions require evaluation and decision.

2. Collect and clarify all data. You need information and guidance to answer the questions "How should I introduce myself?" and "How should I address Mrs. Glotz?" Some hospitals have written policies or practice guidelines about how physicians, nurses, medical students, and residents are to introduce themselves to patients and how patients are to be addressed. If you are unaware of these policies or guidelines, your responsibility is to become informed about what they prescribe or recommend. In many hospitals, however, there are no policies or guidelines to follow.

3. Identify the decision maker. When there are no written policies or guidelines, the choice of how to introduce yourself to Mrs. Glotz and how to address her clearly falls to you.

4. Specify all options. Possible ways to begin the interview are these:

- Introduce yourself as "*Dr.* Sims" or as "Jean Sims, your *doctor*"
- Introduce yourself as "Jean" or "Jean Sims"
- Do not introduce yourself
- Introduce yourself as "Jean Sims, a medical student"

You can address Mrs. Glotz in these ways:

- Glotz
- Mrs. Glotz

- Edith
- "Dear" or other intimate terms

5. Evaluate the options. The moral rules and values that apply to the options you have to initiate the interview with Mrs. Glotz include (a) respect other people, (b) be honest and truthful to your patients, and (c) do not harm your patients. These rules and values tell you the options of no introduction, introduction as Dr. Sims, introduction by first and/or last name with "your doctor" added, and introduction by first name alone are inappropriate. These options either are disrespectful to Mrs. Glotz or leave the impression that she is indeed being interviewed by "a licensed doctor." Furthermore, both legal and moral precedents indicate that Mrs. Glotz has a "right to know" who is interviewing and touching her.

However, there is a possible negative effect of identifying yourself as a medical student. Mrs. Glotz may not feel confident in you nor be open with you. Or she may insist that "a real doctor" examine her. These possible negative effects must be weighed against the positive effect of honesty and forthrightness. If you choose to identify yourself as a medical student, you should have backup plans to handle any negative reactions.

To decide how to address Mrs. Glotz, the moral values of respect for persons and do no harm to the patient rule out the options of *not addressing* Mrs. Glotz directly, *addressing her only by her first or last name,* or addressing her by intimate or colloquial expressions, such as "Dear" or "Dearie." But because you have not met Mrs. Glotz, you are uncertain exactly how you should address her. You could ask her son how she wishes to be addressed (if he is available), or perhaps, you could ask her nurse how Mrs. Glotz prefers to be addressed. But the most efficient way is to ask Mrs. Glotz directly. She is conscious and able to communicate.

6. Select and act on an option.

> You walk into Mrs. Glotz's room. In another era, Edith Glotz would be described as a washerwoman. Her face is deeply creased, and her hands are large and soft as if they must have been scrubbing what? Floors? Clothing? She is leaning heavily against the raised hospital bed. Her face is tense with anxiety. You observe that her ankles are badly swollen. It seems that the oxygen she is receiving via the nasal cannula is helping her.

You introduce yourself: "Hello, I am Jean Sims, a medical student. Dr. Brown wants me to ask you a few questions about how you feel, what happened to you, and what medical problems you had in the past. Shall I call you Mrs. Glotz, or do you prefer I call you by your first name?"

Mrs. Glotz responds in a barely audible heavily accented voice: "Everyone calls me Edy."

"OK. Edy, let me adjust your oxygen tube so you are more comfortable."

She is very anxious. You try to calm her by using a reassuring tone of voice and stroking her hand. This seems to be effective. Her breathing becomes regular, and she is able to answer questions. You begin taking her medical history.

She is a previously healthy 73-year-old nonsmoker. She tells you that after she returned from her husband's funeral yesterday evening, she felt dizzy and nauseous. When she lay down to rest, she began to feel pains in her chest and arms. She took two adult aspirin and went to bed. Her night was restless, but she waited until morning to call her son. Her son brought her to the community hospital ER near her home. When the doctors told her and her son that she had experienced a heart attack, her son insisted that she be transferred to University Hospital where he is an employee. She admits to having a "slight cold" in the past week and some arthritic symptoms in her hands. Just as you finish taking her history Dr. Brown walks into the room.

He tells Mrs. Glotz, "I'm here to help Ms. Sims do a physical examination. We want to make you feel better."

After you listen to her chest, take her pulse, and palpate her abdomen, Dr. Brown comes to the bedside and asks Mrs. Glotz to sit up. "Please lean forward. I want to listen to your lungs. Take a deep breath. Hold it please." Mrs. Glotz breathes deeply. "OK. You can breath normally now." A pause. And again, "Take another deep breath and hold it." Mrs. Glotz breathes deeply a second time. "Ah! Just as I suspected. You have some edema in your lungs." Mrs. Glotz's face freezes with fear, and she asks in a soft voice, "Is that bad?" Dr. Brown says, " We can fix it. You'll be fine." He beckons to you to leave the room with him. You are surprised that Dr. Brown has not answered Mrs. Glotz's question. What should you do?

Analysis

1. Recognize the ethical moment. Mrs. Glotz asks for an explanation of a medical term and an interpretation of her symptoms. The question seems to be very important to Mrs. Glotz, but Dr. Brown merely assures her that she will improve. Should you intervene or accept Dr. Brown's decision to ignore her question? Several factors come into play to cause you some anxiety. You are a student who is learning how to interact with patients. If you question Dr. Brown's action, you may give him the impression that you are challenging his judgment and his authority. Yet it seems to you that Mrs. Glotz's question should be answered. You are facing an ethical moment: Should you intervene or merely follow Dr. Brown's lead?

2. Identify the decision maker. But Dr. Brown, not you, is the responsible decision maker for Mrs. Glotz's care; you are a student. You have no direct responsibility for Mrs. Glotz's care. Dr. Brown's nonanswer may cause her to imagine she has a serious problem, such as cancer, emphysema, and so on. It seems obvious to you that she is not satisfied with Dr. Brown's response but is either reluctant to or incapable of drawing Dr. Brown's attention to her question. What should you do?

3. Identify and evaluate all options. Your options are these:

- To do nothing
- To answer Mrs. Glotz's question yourself
- To ask Dr. Brown outside of Mrs. Glotz's room to explain his response
- To draw Dr. Brown's attention to the question

To do nothing seems inappropriate because lack of information may in fact be harmful to Mrs. Glotz. Furthermore, it seems to you that Mrs. Glotz has a right to information about her diagnosis and treatment. However, if you answer Mrs. Glotz's question, you place yourself in jeopardy with Dr. Brown because you would be answering a question directed to him.

To ask Dr. Brown later about his decision would be presumptuous. Your question would presume that Dr. Brown consciously ignored Mrs. Glotz's question. In fact, he may not have heard her question, or he may have been distracted or even did not understand her question because of her heavy accent. Your inquiry could cause Dr. Brown some embarrassment that could spill over into anger toward you. And yet, Mrs. Glotz has a moral and legal right to a truthful answer from Dr. Brown. What should you do?

4. Select an option and act on it. The best option, in this case, is to draw Dr. Brown's attention to Mrs. Glotz's question in a diplomatic fashion. You might say, "Dr. Brown, I think Mrs. Glotz has a question." If he in fact did not hear or did not understand the question, your intervention would give him the opportunity to translate *edema* and to explain how it is causing some of her symptoms. If he chooses not to explain his diagnosis to Mrs. Glotz, you have fulfilled your responsibility to draw his attention to the question. Later, you can ask why he chose not to respond to Mrs. Glotz.

> You say to Dr. Brown, "Dr. Brown, I think Mrs. Glotz has a question for you."
> Dr. Brown turns back into the room and asks Mrs. Glotz, "Is there something you want to know?" She asks him again: "Is edema good or bad?"
> Dr. Brown explains. "Edema means you have some fluid in your lungs. The fluid is making it hard for you to breathe. We will give you some medicine that should take away some of the fluid."
> "Thank you, doctor."
> In the corridor outside Mrs. Glotz's room, Dr. Brown turns to you and says, "Thanks for alerting me. I did not hear her ask the question. My hearing is not as good as it used to be."

The Lady and the Skinhead

Time: The present
Place: A large community hospital
Cast of characters:

Gerald Blair, M.D., an OB/GYN physician **to be played by YOU**
Lucy Barnes, a patient
Kevin Barnes, Lucy's husband
Anne Bennet, RN, Lucy's nurse
James Burroughs, Ph.D., a clinical ethicist

It is a terrible case. One you will always remember. Lucy Barnes, a lovely 30-year-old woman, is dying. Only four weeks ago, she came to you because she was experiencing vaginal bleeding. You remember your first impression: a simply dressed elegant woman. Your impressions were jarred when you discovered that she had several tattoos on her torso. Yet when she received the diagnosis, she conducted herself with the poise of a lady. Now she is in a coma, dying from a virulent ovarian cancer.

As you walk toward the conference room, you review the conversation you had with Anne Bennet, Lucy's nurse, that prompted a meeting with her husband. Anne told you that Kevin, Lucy's husband, whom you have not met, caused a disturbance in Lucy's room. "Dr. Blair, Lucy's husband insists that everything be done to keep her alive. He's a Skinhead with a Nazi swastika tattooed on each arm. I think he is sadistic!!"

Anne's report disturbs you because you know that aggressive therapy is last thing you want to do. Lucy cannot recover from this cancer; it has spread throughout her abdominal cavity. If only Lucy had prepared a living will or durable power of attorney for health care decisions before she went into the coma. But the reality is that she lost consciousness before this could be discussed.

Analysis

1. What kind of problem is this? This is an ethical dilemma. There is a conflict between your duty to do no harm to Lucy (therapy would only prolong her dying) and your duty to respect the authority of her surrogate decision maker, her husband Kevin. You and Kevin appear to be on opposite sides of the question of limiting or stopping therapy. You cannot fulfill both obligations simultaneously.

2. Clarify and collect all data. This case is complex. Its complexity must be unraveled before judgment and decision making can occur. All your information about Kevin and his demands is secondhand. You see Kevin through the eyes of Anne Bennet, Lucy's nurse. Your first responsibility is to assess Kevin and find out what Kevin is demanding. Clarification can happen only if you meet with Kevin face-to-face. Before meeting with Kevin, you must examine your own feelings about Anne Bennet's description of Kevin as a "Skinhead." Negative images of violence, prejudice, and terror are linked in your mind with the word *Skinhead*. There is a real danger that your negative feelings about Skinheads will intrude into your conversation with Kevin. You realize that one way to protect against the danger of confrontation with Kevin is to invite a neutral party, such as the hospital's ethics consultant, to organize and lead the meeting with Kevin.

3. Identify the decision maker. You realize that the question of who should make this decision is very much in contention. Lucy Barnes has not made her desires known by legal document, and she never discussed her end-of-life wishes with you. Her husband is the surrogate decision maker, but it has been reported that he desires what you believe is unreasonable and cruel.

4. Specify all options.

Jim Burroughs, the clinical ethicist, meets you at the conference room door. He introduces you to Kevin. Kevin, indeed, has a shaved head, an earring, and tattoos. Jim informs you that Kevin is a musician who is becoming more and more known for his contemporary music. Jim asks you to review Lucy's medical condition and the history of her cancer. As you relay the sobering information, you notice that tears are flowing down Kevin's cheeks. Jim asks whether Kevin wishes to take a break, but he insists that you finish your analysis. When you finish, Jim asks your opinion about Lucy's future and the types of therapy available to treat her. You are straightforward in your answers.

"There is no hope for recovery. I recommend that only comfort care be provided so that Lucy's suffering will be shortened."

Jim then asks Kevin to express his feelings about Lucy's predicament. Kevin's response reveals his deep love for Lucy and his fear of losing her. Several times Kevin addresses you directly. "Dr. Blair, are you sure there is no hope? Has the cancer gone too far? Could you be wrong?"

He clings to the hope that Lucy may recover. Your heart sinks because you feel that a confrontation is coming. Kevin wants "everything done," and you are convinced that therapy should be stopped. You are about to express your feelings when Jim intervenes.

"Thank you, Dr. Blair and Mr. Barnes, for so clearly and coura-geously stating your positions. It would be unfortunate if we allowed this discussion to become a battle of wills that forgets the reason for our meeting. We are meeting because Lucy cannot tell us what she desires. We must remember that our decisions about Lucy's care should reflect what Lucy would desire if she could express them. We cannot allow our personal and professional desires to override her wishes. Unfortunately, Lucy cannot give us directions."

"Kevin, I sense that you cannot bear the thought of making a mis-take in judgment if you would agree to stop Lucy's therapy. You know how much Lucy enjoyed life, and you are not sure that she would want to stop therapy. Also, I sense that Dr. Blair feels strongly that he would be violating his responsibility as a physician to do no harm to Lucy by continuing aggressive therapy that he judges is futile."

"I would like to suggest a third option," Dr. Burroughs continues. "A decision can be delayed until a second opinion can be gotten. Kevin, would you feel more comfortable about agreeing to stopping therapy if a second opinion by another physician agrees with Dr. Blair's?" Kevin nods his head. "Dr. Blair, are you willing to continue therapy until another oncologist can examine Lucy and give us his thoughts about continuing or discontinuing therapy?"

"Yes," you say. "I think that is a good plan."

5. *Evaluate and act on the options.* Both options (to stop or to continue therapy) are supported by ethical values. Your medical assessment and experience sup-port your recommendation to stop therapy because you do not want to harm Lucy. Mr. Barnes's knowledge of his wife's attitudes toward her life and death, his deep love, and his responsibility for Lucy, as well as his uncertainty about the diagnosis and prognosis support continuation of therapy because he feels he must be confident that he has made the right decision. Because of this impasse, the clinical ethicist suggests a compromise third option. He recommends that a second opinion be gotten and that until this opinion is gotten, the therapeutic course be continued. If the second opinion is the same as the first opinion, Dr. Burroughs feels that Mr. Barnes's need to be certain when he agrees to stop the therapy is indeed the right thing, the loving act, for his wife and himself. The third option asks that both you and Kevin concede something and still preserve your dignity.

The Schoolboy and the
Board of Education

Time: The present
Place: A doctor's office
Cast of characters:

George Stevens, M.D., a family practice doctor **to be played by YOU**
Charles "Charlie" Evans, a 17-year-old patient
Jane and Chester Evans, Charles's parents

You are curious and a bit puzzled as you walk toward your office after examining the day's last patient. Your secretary, Sarah, scheduled
a meeting with Charlie Evans and his parents. Sarah told you the
Evanses called while you were seeing patients and would not specify
the reason for the meeting but said it is very important that you meet
with them today. You wonder what this is all about. Charlie's illness is
progressing, but he has been relatively stable all summer.

Charlie has been your patient since his birth to Jane and Chester.
Chester is a prominent local farmer, and Jane has a thriving antiques/
collectibles business. They are good parents with the financial and
personal resources needed to care for Charlie. At an early age, Charlie developed symptoms of progressive muscular weakness that
prompted you to refer him for diagnosis to Dr. Bevens, pediatric neurologist, at the state medical school. The diagnosis was muscular dystrophy. You have managed his care since his diagnosis.

Despite the poor prognosis and progressive paralysis, Charlie and
his parents determined he would live his life to the fullest possible extent. You are very proud of Charlie because he is a living example of
how a person can successfully face a tragic illness when he or she has
a supportive family and community. Charlie and his parents have accepted and put into practice the best medical advice about treating
the muscular dystrophy's symptoms. The Evans family, especially
Charlie, has studied scientific literature on muscular dystrophy and
are probably better informed than you are about the status of scientific information about muscular dystrophy's etiology, natural history,
and therapy. The enthusiastic support of his parents and siblings as

well as his schoolmates helped Charlie to excel. Charlie is the state high school chess champion, and he has carried a 3.5 average despite his being wheelchair bound. He is entering his senior year in two weeks. You wonder what the agenda is for this meeting.

"Hi Charlie, Jane, Chester. Good to see you. Sarah told me that this is an important meeting. Can you tell me what it's all about? Have you found a new study on muscular dystrophy?"

Jane responds: "No, Dr. Stevens. I wish we did find something encouraging. We asked to meet with you because we need your help on a matter that is very important to Charlie and to us."

"Well, of course, I'll help you the best I can."

Chester enters the conversation by telling you, "Dr. Stevens, we think Charlie should explain why we are here. He has convinced us that we need your opinion and help."

Charlie uses his electronic controls to position his wheelchair so that he faces you directly. "Dr. Stevens, you know I am about to begin my senior year at Bufton High. I really look forward to this year. But I know that my muscular dystrophy has progressed more rapidly in the past year. My breathing is becoming more and more difficult."

"You have been very honest with me about my future. I really appreciate that. I know, and you know, that eventually the muscular dystrophy will overwhelm my chest muscles and I will not be able to breathe." Charlie pauses. "I do not want to live on a ventilator."

You say, "Charlie, let's cross that bridge when we come to it. It may be a long time before you need a ventilator."

Charlie politely but firmly responds, "I would like to discuss this now and not postpone it."

"All right. What do you have in mind?"

Charlie looks at his parents, who nod encouragement to him, and then turns back to you. "I am asking you to write a letter to Mr. Taft (president of the Bufton Board of Education) that I am not to be resuscitated if I have a respiratory arrest while I'm at school."

"Charlie, your request is a real surprise. I will need to think this over before I can decide whether to do what you ask."

"I didn't expect you to answer me today," Charlie comments.

"OK, Charlie. Let me ask a few questions before we leave today. Chester and Jane, do you agree with Charlie's request?"

"Yes, we do," Jane responds.

Chester adds: "We had a long talk with Charlie about this. We also talked to our minister, Pastor Eccles. He supports Charlie's request. This is not an impulsive act by Charlie or us. We love Charlie and do not wish to lose him. But as you have told us, there is no hope in sight for recovery from muscular dystrophy. It is Charlie's life, and he should have a say in how it ends." Jane nods her head in approval.

"Charlie, can I ask you why you do not want to be dependent on a ventilator?"

Charlie quickly responds, "I still remember having that tube in my throat when I had that bad case of pneumonia a couple of years ago. I hated it. I couldn't talk. I couldn't move. I couldn't eat. And it hurt!"

"Well, you have made your feelings clear. I cannot argue with your experience. But may I ask you and your parents whether you have consulted with Dr. Bevens (the pediatric neurologist) about your request?"

"No, we have not. We think you are in a better position to help us than he is."

"Thank you for your confidence in me. What I meant to ask is whether you have consulted with Dr. Bevens about your chances for respiratory failure and the current technology for ventilator support? You were examined by him last spring. Am I correct?"

"Yes, but we did not ask him those questions."

This request stuns you. Charlie is asking you to write DNR (do not resuscitate) instructions for the Board of Education and Bufton High. Should you agree to do this? Should you disagree? What should you do?

Analysis

1. What kind of problem is this? Charlie's request raises questions that go far beyond your professional responsibility to respond to Charlie's desire not to be placed on a ventilator. More is at stake than the DNR order. His request raises questions about the extent and limitations of your community role and responsibility to the community. If you agree to write a letter to the school board, the board would face an unprecedented choice: to follow your instructions that would oblige Charlie's instructors and high school officials to act contrary to their ingrained obligations to save a student's life if it is in jeopardy or to refuse to honor Charlie's request to die. Charlie's request creates an individual and social ethics dilemma.

2. Collect and clarify all data. There are many unknowns and unanswered questions that you need to identify and clarify before you can decide what to do.

3. Identify the decision maker. Technically, Charlie is still a minor who is obviously dependent on his parents. But because his parents support Charlie's request, the question of who should make the decision whether to be resuscitated is moot. Both Charlie and his parents have the moral authority, if not legal authority, to decide against resuscitation and ventilator dependency. However, you alone must make a decision whether you will write a letter to the school board in support of Charlie's request. What should you do?

4. Specify and evaluate all options. As you converse with Charlie and his parents, you realize that you have both short-range and long-range options. The long-range options mean that short-range you will need to temporize. However, sooner or later you will decide whether to write the letter. Your short-range options include the following:

- Refuse to write the letter
- Agree to write the letter
- Refer the decision to Dr. Bevens, the pediatric neurologist
- Temporize the decision until you get more clarity
- Call Mr. Taft, the Board of Education president
- Call your attorney for an opinion about Charlie as decision maker

You could wash your hands of the matter and refuse to write the letter. But you would injure Charlie's and his parents' trust in you. Also, refusal would be disrespectful of both Charlie and his parents because they have thought carefully about this request.

You could agree to write the letter, but there are too many unanswered matters and the implications of this decision are far-reaching. You, Charlie, and his parents are not the only ones who would be affected by your agreeing to write this letter. Your decision would put severe burdens on the Board of Education members, Charlie's instructors, and the high school officials.

You could recommend that Charlie revisit Dr. Bevens and ask him to write the letter. But that would be passing the burden of choice on to Dr. Bevens, who has been involved in Charlie's care primarily as a consultant. But you could recommend that Charlie ask Dr. Bevens for more prognostic and technical information. However, you are better prepared to gather and evaluate this information. You can contact Bevens by conference call and have Charlie and his parents present.

You could call Mr. Taft (Board of Education president) but to what purpose? It would be inappropriate to pass the decision on to him and his board. But it would be useful to inform him that you are facing this choice and need to know what his (and his board's) reaction would be to such a proposal. This would be a politically wise action, but it certainly does not resolve your dilemma.

Calling your attorney to ask his opinion about how the legal system would regard a decision like this by a technically minor person is a wise choice. It is important that you have information about the legal implications of writing such a letter. You would obtain legal advice, but the decision would still be yours.

The best short-range option is to temporize. Obviously, you cannot make a decision at this moment because there are still many unexplored issues.

You also have some long-range options: After you have gathered more information from your lawyer, the president of the school board, and Dr. Bevens and after Charlie and his parents have received Dr. Bevens's opinion about the course of Charlie's disease as well as the latest scientific and therapeutic developments, you will be better prepared to make a decision.

The moral principles that support your writing the letter are the free choice made by Charlie and his parents not to undergo a potentially life-saving intervention, resuscitation, and ventilator support. Furthermore, their choice of not using these interventions would benefit other persons who could need these interventions. However, this choice is not made in a vacuum. This choice would affect many other persons. It is unseemly to impose Charlie's free choice on others by your letter. You cannot and should not force other autonomous persons to act contrary to their beliefs and convictions, as well as to established social behavior. Your letter would cause a stir among the board members that would probably ripple out to the community through gossip and media attraction to the novelty of the request. This would negatively affect your practice because you would be asked to meet with the media.

Nonetheless, if you are convinced that Charlie's request is legitimate, you have the option of engaging in a long-range and arduous campaign to convince the school board and the community that not to resuscitate Charlie would be a morally and legally responsible action.

In any event, this decision demands that you obtain help and counsel from knowledgeable and experienced persons from the helping professions, the legal profession, and the community. The next chapter explores how you can obtain help when you face an unprecedented or unusual dilemma.

Any Port in a Storm?

How and Where to Find Help

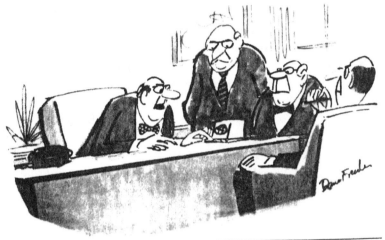

Miss Dugan, will you send someone in here who can distinguish right from wrong?'

Mrs. Olson's request to die from an overdose of morphine ("Please Help Me!" p. 19) compels Dr. Byrn to ask a senior physician for help. Dr. Braun's response, "Welcome to the profession," does not help him sort out his options and responsibilities, but it clearly reminds him that to be a physician means that he must make difficult, sometimes lonely, choices.

Dr. Braun's response points out the harsh reality of your physician role. The license to practice medicine frees you in many ways, and it also burdens you. You are free from legal sanctions to prescribe and give drugs as part of your patients' therapy. You may explore confidential and intimate information about your patients' behavior to facilitate your diagnosis and therapy. During physical examinations, you see and touch your patients' unclothed bodies with impunity. However, your freedom to perform these and other actions is balanced by significant burdens. You must make diagnostic and therapeutic choices that affect your patients' quality of life and, in many cases, their length of life. And you are held accountable by law for any negative sequelae of your decisions.

Although your medical education and clinical training equip you with knowledge and skills to make diagnostic and therapeutic decisions, you are never fully prepared to meet the challenges of clinical predicaments and dilemmas. Clinical ethics cases are "minidramas" in which you are a central character who possesses power and has major responsibilities. What you do or do not do and what you say or do not say profoundly influence the patient, family, institution, and the outcome of the case.

The cases presented in this book are abstract stories that do not and cannot capture the emotions and tumult of a clinical ethics predicament. Your patients and their families are confused, angry, anxious, fearful, denying, and grief-stricken. You also feel strong emotions: sympathy, antipathy, anger, impatience, compassion, distance, fear, confidence, frustration. Furthermore hovering in the background of each case are other professionals (nurses, technicians, chaplains, administrators, lawyers, accountants, peers, etc.) who stand like a Greek chorus ready to comment on your performance. All contribute a special brand of stress. When the emotional storm of a clinical predicament swirls around you, where do you turn for help? You need to consult with someone. Your training instinctively points you toward the harbor of second opinions.

Traditional Consultation Models

Curbside Consultations

From your first day on rounds, you and your colleagues learn a very important practice guideline: "CYA." This slightly vulgar acronym ("Cover your ass") reminds you always to take steps to protect yourself, especially when there are perplexing questions about a patient's diagnosis or therapy. Getting the opinion and/or advice of another physician is indeed a CYA action. Second opinions also give you another set of eyes through which you view the clinical puzzle. In many cases, second opinions confirm your judgment, and at other times they give you new insights that prompt you to rethink your diagnosis,

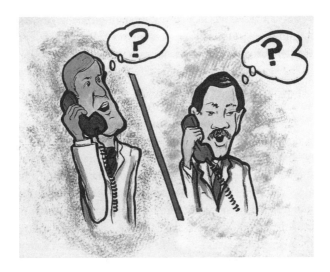

your therapy, or both. The CYA practice guideline tells you, "When in doubt, obtain a second opinion either through direct referrals to a colleague or through curbside consultations by paging or phoning a colleague for advice."

The importance of the CYA rule and the value of having access to trusted advisers prompts you to create your network of advisers. Your address file is filled with pager and phone numbers of colleagues, mentors, acquaintances, and professors who become your informal network of advisers whom you call on for advice when facing a perplexing diagnostic or therapeutic problem. It is not unusual for you to ask these same advisers for advice when the perplexing clinical problem is ethical rather than medical. Dr. Byrn's question to Dr. Braun (p. 19) is clearly ethical: Should he or should he not overdose Mrs. Olson?

As your practice grows, you expand your informal network of advisers to include other professionals. You include nurses who see clinical ethics predicaments from different perspectives and who witness both effective and ineffective ways of resolving them. Your network has at least one lawyer, perhaps a friend of a friend, who gives practical advice about protecting yourself when you face these perplexing questions. Sometimes you call a minister, imam, or rabbi for advice concerning your patient's or your own religious beliefs and ask how these apply to your dilemma. Nonetheless, trusted colleagues, especially your medical school and residency friends, are the advisers you call most frequently. However, unless your colleagues are prepared by special education and training in clinical ethics decision making, the advice you receive in these curbside consultations reflects their personal moral perspectives and experiences rather than a broader view of the moral demands of practicing medicine.

Institutional Consultation Models

All hospitals and health care organizations institutionalize and expand the harbor of second opinions. Instead of one-to-one consultations, institutional models rely on the collective advice of physicians either in regularly scheduled staff meetings or on a case-by-case basis. Some of these institutional consultations are postfactum peer reviews—for example, the M&M (morbidity and mortality) conference; some are proactive group consultations—for example, the patient management conference (PMC). At the M&M conference, you report your patients' diseases, complications, and deaths. Your colleagues' questions and critiques, for the most part, concentrate on the thoroughness of your data collection, judgment, decisions, and patient management. Although the M&M conference can be painful, it does provide peer review of your judgments and decisions that assists you in future cases.

The PMC, on the other hand, is a proactive forum for testing options or for choosing strategies to implement treatment decisions for a specific patient. The PMC usually involves a broad spectrum of health care professionals that ranges from physicians to social workers. The value of the PMC is that it provides a forum for open discussion and exploration of options and opinions prior to making decisions, choosing strategies, or both.

Usually, these institutional models offer advice and critiques on medical questions, but they also examine and critique the way you handle ethical questions raised by your report. However, institutional models have the same limitations as individual curbside consultations. The feedback you receive reflects the personal and professional experiences of the physicians and other health care professionals who participate in the conference rather than a broader view of the moral requirements of practicing medicine. A broader view of the moral requirements of your practice is important because each case places you in the intersection of professional, religious, and ethnic moral positions and assumptions. You find yourself in a "pluralism" (the coexistence of a number of often conflicting moral rules). You, your patient, family members, and other health care professionals bring their moral beliefs with them when they enter the case. Pluralism may contribute to or cause the clinical predicament. Resolution of the clinical predicament requires a perspective based on more than medical opinion.

Legal Consultation Model

The importance of obtaining more than medical advice on clinical predicaments leads hospitals and health care institutions to expand the institutional models of consultation to include legal consultation. In fact, many hospitals and health care institutions require you to consult with a health care lawyer before you make decisions in neonatal and pediatric cases. Legal consultations are highly refined and institutionalized CYA consultations. The health care lawyer's primary function is to protect you and the hospital from lawsuits and legal sanctions. However, because legal and ethical traditions address the same questions (e.g., freedom, informed consent, do no harm, compensation for harm, fairness, etc.), health care lawyers also frequently comment on ethical as well as legal ramifications of a case. Case law and ethics are so interwoven that it is very difficult to separate the two. Careful distinction between legal and ethical questions will help you when you seek advice from an attorney. The ethical choice may not always be the legal choice.

Nontraditional Consultation Models

Recognition of the need to expand the view of clinical responsibilities beyond the medical and legal perspective leads to the formation of nontraditional models of consultation. Nontraditional models include (a) health care ethics policies (HCEPs), (b) health care ethics committees (HCECs), (c) health care ethics consultation services (HCECSs), (d) clinical ethics departments (CEDs) and (e) organizational ethics consultation (OEC).

Health Care Ethics Policies (HCEPs)

Many health care organizations develop HCEP and procedural guidelines to assist patients, families, and physicians in clinical ethics predicaments. When you join a health care organization, ask for a copy of the institution's clinical ethics policies. The availability of these policies indicates that the institution has a position on issues of patient rights, the responsibilities of their health care professionals, and the social responsibilities of the institution. These policies give you an understanding of the institution's commitments and show you exactly how the institution has created procedures, services, and other resources that you can rely on when you have need for consultation.

A comprehensive HCEP handbook will address common clinical ethics predicaments and include the institution's positions and procedures concerning
the following:

- Do not resuscitate orders (DNR)
- Withholding/withdrawing life support
- Brain death (definition and diagnostic tests)
- Patient refusal of treatment
- Nutritional support (providing or removing)
- Confidentiality and truth telling
- Research ethics (informed consent)
- Conflict of interest (physicians and industry)
- Reproductive ethics (abortion, birth control, assisted reproduction)
- Refusal to treat (moral conflict with participation in certain therapies)
- Care of the terminally ill patient

The best policies include descriptive definitions of critical concepts, such as
brain death, resuscitation procedures, and so on, as well as practical guidelines
to follow and resources to call on when you experience conflict in the management of a case or when you have questions about your responsibilities.

Health Care Ethics Committee (HCEC)

Frequently, HCEPs refer to a HCEC as a resource you can access when you
need ethics advice. The mission of the HCEC is to provide clinical ethics advice to the institution and its staff. Usually, the HCEC is composed of both
medical and nonmedical professionals, as well as community representatives.
The interdisciplinary membership of the HCEC provides a perspective on clinical ethics issues that goes beyond the medical and legal. Although the HCEC's
function differs from institution to institution, generally they provide all or
some of the following services to the institution and to you. They serve as policy advisers to the hospital administration. In fact, many ethics policies are
developed in the HCEC and presented as practice guidelines for the health
care institution. The HCEC also has a dual education role. It provides self-
education in medical ethics to HCEC committee members and organizes insti-
tution-wide education in clinical ethics for physicians, nurses, health care
technicians, and others. Finally, the HCEC provides an ethics consultation
service to staff members, nurses, patients, and families. The HCEC's consulta-

tive service is provided in one of two ways. The HCEC assembles as an entire committee to meet with you, your patient, and/or family members to discuss the predicament, or it has on-call "ethics consultation teams" to provide ethics consultation at the bedside.

These different forms of consultation have pluses and minuses. The full-committee consultative service does provide a broad spectrum of ethics advice, but its size (usually large) and its formal setting (in a conference room with a chairman and committee members) can be slow in convening, cumbersome in operation, and threatening to patients and family members. The HCEC ethics consult team is a smaller version of the full committee and thus suffers some of the limitations mentioned above, but the team does go to the bedside and is available on call. The team service is more efficient and user-friendly.

Clinical Ethics Department (CED)

Clinical ethics departments are being established in hospitals and health care institutions. The members of a CED come from a variety of professional backgrounds and are educated and trained in clinical ethics consultation. The presence of a CED in a health care institution indicates the institution's commitment to making ethics advice available to its staff members, patients, and families. The CED expands the traditional curbside consultation model to include clinical ethics consultants. When the CED staff is incorporated into daily clinical activities, their advice is informed with the intellectual, emotional, and organizational realities of making clinical decisions. Not infrequently, CED members also serve on the HCEC. They provide education for the members of the HCEC and use the HCEC as a forum for review of their consultations as well as a forum for discussion of policy and procedural issues.

A fully developed CED provides ethics advice and education to the professional and administrative staff of the health care institution in a variety of ways:

- Providing on-call ethics consultation
- Attending daily patient care rounds
- Leading clinical ethics patient care rounds
- Providing ethics in-service seminars and lectures
- Providing continuing medical education seminars on clinical ethics topics
- Establishing clinical ethics journal clubs

Organizational Ethics Consultation (OEC)

Finally, a more recent development in institutional ethics consultation is the development of OEC groups. These groups are designed to provide advice concerning the health care institution's positions and behavior toward individual patients, providers, and employees and toward the communities served by the health care institution as well as by other medical and nonmedical institutions. Although in its infancy, the OEC has the potential to become a major resource for finance, patient management, insurance, and other issues that arise in the interface between medicine and business.

A Final Note

There are several national organizations devoted to promoting understanding of the humanistic and ethical aspects of medical care and to encouraging the development of skilled clinical ethics consultants. These groups range from think tanks such as the Hastings Center to national organizations. In 1998, three of these national organizations (the Society for Health and Human Values, the Society for Bioethics Consultation, and the American Association of Bioethics) organized into one national organization, the American Society for Bioethics and Humanities.

One of the first publications produced by the merger of the three organizations was the Report of the Task Force on Standards for Bioethics Consultation, *Core Competencies for Health Care Consultation*.[1] This report is the result of two years of work by 21 scholars and clinicians in the fields of health care ethics, policy, and patient care. In addition to the report's description of the core competencies needed for a person or committee to offer clinical ethics consultation, the report contains a bibliography and a listing of academic departments, bioethics centers, regional networks, and other organizations that contributed substantive materials and curricula to the task force. The report is a valuable resource to those interested in pursuing a career in clinical ethics or wishing to expand their knowledge of clinical ethics.

Conclusion

The tradition of medicine and the expectations of your patients place a heavy burden on you. You must contribute your knowledge and skills to choices made in difficult circumstances with great values at stake. Awareness of and skill in the ethics of practicing medicine will make you more sensitive both to your needs and the needs of your patients and their families. To meet your patients' ethical and human needs as well as their need for scientific analysis and action means that your education in the science of medicine and the ethics of medicine must continue throughout your professional career. Challenge your colleagues as they gather at scientific and professional meetings to give time to discuss the moral and humanistic dimensions of their practice that will be eternally the true measure of caring for the sick.

Note

1. *Core Competencies for Health Care Consultation* is available from the American Society of Bioethics and Humanities, 4700 W. Lake, Glenview, IL 60025-1485; phone (847) 375-4725; fax (847) 375-6345. For additional helpful information, visit the ASBH Website at http://www.asbh.org.

Appendix

Problems in Clinical Ethics

Although there are many ways to categorize clinical ethics problems, I find that linking these problems to your many roles as a physician is the most practical. As a physician, you enter the lives of persons at critical times in their personal history. Physicians, like ministers, are present in persons' lives when they are "hatched, matched, and dispatched."

Patients come to you for information, advice, and care when they face illnesses or critical turning points in their lives. You ask them to be candid, compliant, and observant. They, in turn, expect honesty, loyalty, and compassion from you. A physician-patient relationship is formed built on trust and mutual understanding of the roles played by the participants. During this relationship you take on many roles: adviser, guide, confidant, scientist, counselor, healer, teacher. These roles carry with them responsibilities, duties, and obligations. As noted above, at times, these responsibilities can create problems, clinical predicaments that need solutions.

Physician as Reproduction Adviser

Patients come to you seeking advice and help as they face questions raised by their desire to reproduce. Their requests can introduce ethics questions concerning the following:

- *Genetic counseling* (amniocentesis, family history of recessive/dominant genetic defects, etc.)
- *Reproductive technology* (in vitro fertilization, surrogate motherhood, artificial insemination by donor, embryo transfer, egg donation, etc.)
- *Unwanted/unexpected pregnancies* (abortion, sterilization as contraceptive means, sterilization of the psychologically challenged, etc.)

Physician as Confidant

In the course of your clinical encounters, you may ask personal questions about a patient's lifestyle to assist your analysis of symptoms and to give advice. Patients may volunteer intimate information, or you may gain it by happenstance or deduction. The giving and receiving of intimate information creates the obligation of confidentiality. The obligation to retain confidences can raise serious predicaments for you when they clash with other duties and responsibilities. These predicaments include the following:

- *The duty to warn* innocent third parties (e.g., a spouse who is not aware of her husband's HIV status)
- *The duty to disclose* information to third parties who have a legitimate interest in this information (e.g., a medical condition that has the potential to cause serious problems while driving or working)
- *Justification for deception* when asked for confidential information by parties who do not have a legitimate interest
- *Disclosure of diagnostic and therapeutic information* to employers, insurance companies, and so on

Physician as Gatekeeper

Deciding who will receive therapy or what level of therapy has always been part of the physician's role. However, economic changes are creating an unparalleled "gatekeeper" role for physicians. You face decisions about allocation of benefits (medical resources) and burdens (denial of expensive or experimental therapies) for your patients. Questions of justice raise important ethical questions, such as these:

- Rationing limited medical resources
- Managing triage in times of disaster
- Procuring of organs for transplantation

- Listing patients for transplantation
- Distributing organs for transplantation

Physician as Scientist

Patients provide the raw material for scientific research into the effectiveness of drugs, procedures, and the like. Drug companies, university centers of medical research, and government agencies want physicians to participate in research projects. The pressure to contribute to the advancement of scientific knowledge and its application to clinical problems can raise serious questions for you:

- *Informed consent* (taking the time and energy to communicate what your patient is required to do as well as the risks and benefits of participating in a research study)
- *Manipulation of consent* (using persuasive powers to convince patients to participate without their voluntary consent)
- *Therapeutic innovations versus experimentation* (are your treatments therapeutic innovations or experimental procedures?)
- *Obligations to participate in research* for the benefit of society versus the benefit to individual patients

Physician as Decision Maker

The power and responsibility that you have as a decision maker raises serious questions about the specific exercise of your power. The following can produce clinical predicaments or dilemmas:

- *Paternalism* (making decisions for competent persons without their approval)
- Patients with *unusual beliefs or irrational choices*
- *Determination of patients' competency* or the lack of competency
- *Children and adolescent assent* or consent
- *Intellectually and emotionally challenged adults*

Physician as Guide at End-of-Life

Because you are dedicated to preserving and enhancing your patients' lives, the assistance they ask from you as they face the end of life is most difficult to fulfill. Your responsibilities as guide for end-of-life decisions are complex and involve the following issues:

- Do not resuscitate orders (DNR). When are they appropriate?
- Withdrawal of life-sustaining therapies. When are they appropriate?
- Withholding of life-sustaining therapies. When are they appropriate?
- Definition of futile medical therapy
- The quality of life of your patients
- Euthanasia (active or passive, voluntary or involuntary)
- Physician-assisted suicide
- Brain death
- Persistent vegetative state

Glossary

Advance directives Legal documents that permit competent adults to direct the medical care they wish to receive if they are unable to make their wishes known either through a living will or by appointing a person(s) with the power to serve as the attorney-in-fact for heath care decisions (a durable power of attorney for health care choices).

Autonomy The moral value that holds in high esteem individual freedom (a person's capacity to make self-reliant, independent, individual decisions).

Clinical predicament A complicated, perplexing situation from which it is difficult to disengage oneself that arises in the course of clinical practice.

Durable power of attorney A legal document by which a competent adult names a person(s) to act as his or her attorney-in-fact to make health care decisions if he or she becomes unable to make them for him or herself.

Duty A responsibility, associated with professional status, that requires specific action.

Ethical moment The time in a clinical encounter when the question of obligation, duty, or responsibility occurs.

Ethics Philosophical and/or theological study of morality and the justification of moral rules of conduct and moral values.

Justice The moral value that holds in high esteem the fair distribution of the benefits and burdens of living in society.

Law The sum total of rules and regulations by which a society is governed; the composite of local, state, and federal court decisions, regulations, and procedures.

Life The moral value that holds in high esteem the property or quality of humans, plants, and animals that distinguishes them from inorganic matter or dead organisms.

Living will A legal document by which competent adults can direct the medical care they desire if they become terminally ill and unable to make medical decisions for themselves.

Moral dilemma A clinical predicament whose solution requires a choice between competing obligations.

Moral knowledge A person's understanding, achieved through education, culture, and experience, of duties, responsibilities, and obligations.

Moral quandary A clinical predicament that creates a state of great perplexity and uncertainty because of a lack of moral precedents.

Morality A collection of rules of conduct found in a culture, subculture, religion, or professional group and frequently found gathered in a code of morality (aka, a code of ethics).

Obligation The consequence of assuming a responsibility.

Responsibility Action for which a person is held accountable.

Right(s) A claim, based in tradition or law that a person is empowered to act (positive right) or is to be left undisturbed (negative right).

Rule of conduct A written or unwritten directive for behavior.

Index

About the Author

George A. Kanoti, S.T.D., was born in Lorain, Ohio, and raised in Fontana, California. He is a graduate of St. Louis University and the Catholic University of America. He is Emeritus Staff of the Cleveland Clinic Foundation, Cleveland, Ohio, and the first holder of the F. J. O'Neill Chair of Clinical Bioethics and first chairman of the Department of Bioethics at the Cleveland Clinic. His academic career includes professorships at the Catholic University of America, John Carroll University, and Ohio State University. His clinical career spans more than a decade of providing clinical ethics consultation and assisting health care organizations here and abroad to establish ethics consultation services and ethics committees. He is cofounder of the Society of Bioethics and one of its first presidents. He is a member of the Task Force on Core Competencies for Health Care Ethics Consultation sponsored by the American Society for Bioethics and Humanities. He lectures in the United States, Germany, and Argentina. His publications include articles in the *Encyclopedia of Bioethics,* the *New England Journal of Medicine,* and other professional and academic journals.